The You Book

A Treasury of Health and Healing

Earlyne Chaney, Ph.D.

Astara's Library of
Body/Mind/Spirit Masterworks

Published by

Astara

800 W. Arrow Highway
Upland, CA 91786

Cover Design: Steve Doolittle
Photo: The Image Bank West/Whitney Lane © 1990

Library of Congress Catalogue Card 90-84838
ISBN 0-918936-23-3

Printed in the United States of America

A MESSAGE FROM ASTARA

The publishers of this book have made it available to you in the belief that it will make a contribution to your life on its various important levels: physical, emotional, intellectual, and spiritual.

Actually, we consider this volume to be an extension of the teachings contained in Astara's series of mystical studies known as *Astara's Book of Life*. The lessons comprising the *Book of Life* are distributed on a world-wide basis only to members of Astara. Astara was founded in 1951 as a non-profit religious and educational organization including the following concepts:

1. A center of all religions, oriented to mystical Christianity but accepting and teaching all religions as beneficial to humankind.
2. A school of the ancient Mysteries, offering a compendium of the esoteric teachings of all ages.
3. A fraternity of all philosophies, coordinating many viewpoints of humankind and the interacting inner structures which unite us as one in the infinite.
4. An institute of psychic research, with emphasis on spiritual healing of physical, emotional and mental aspects, and to life before and after physical incarnation.

If these areas of interest are appealing to you, you may wish to pursue the studies of *Astara's Book of Life* as have thousands of others in some ninety countries around the world.

To give you information about Astara, its teachings, and other possible services to you, we have prepared a treatise entitled *Finding Your Place in the Golden Age*. You may have it without cost or obligation. Write:

Other books by Earlyne Chaney

Remembering — The Autobiography of a Mystic
The Masters and Astara
Secrets From Mount Shasta
The Book of Beginning Again
Revelations of Things to Come
Beyond Tomorrow — a Book of Prophecies
Shining Moments of a Mystic
Initiation in the Great Pyramid
Forever Young

- - - - - - - - - - -

Published by Samuel Weiser, Inc.

The Mystery of Death and Dying—
Initiation at the Moment of Death
The Eyes Have It

- - - - - - - - - - -

Astara's Book of Life
A series of esoteric teachings of the
Mystery Schools of all ages

- - - - - - - - - - -

Books in Collaboration

Kundalini and the Third Eye
With William Messick
The Mystical Marriage of Science and Spirit
By Frances Paelian
(Based on the teachings of Earlyne Chaney)

The You Book

A Treasury of Health and Healing

Table of Contents

A Note from the Publisher

The products, remedies, formulas and ideas in this book are not in any way offered as medical advice or prescriptions for the relief or cure of any illness whatsoever. Nor is any diagnosis intended or implied.

Neither author nor publisher intends that the contents of this book replace competent medical advice given by a duly authorized professional. The book reflects the author's personal research and experience which may or may not parallel those of the reader.

Any company's products are more, or less, effective for one person than those of another company. In the final analysis, each person needs to experiment and compare for himself or herself to judge results personally.

Neither author nor publisher receives payment for any product listed or recommended in this book. Inclusion of products and companies was entirely at the discretion of the author and based upon her personal experiences and research.

Chapter One

Humanity Poised – For Power or for Peril

Before beginning this book I decided to assemble information sent me through the years to be used as a basis for writing about *you*. Any writings about *you* should include that which *you* have expressed. I was considering several aspects about you to be included —

1. the health and well-being of your physical body;
2. the influence of your mind in the holistic being;
3. your mind and spirit.

To determine which aspect most appealed to you, and about which you wanted to know more, I sent out a questionnaire covering all three. To my surprise, very few expressed a desire for knowledge concerning the latter two. I was bombarded with questions and information relative to health and well-being. Part of my questionnaire asked about doctor-patient relationship and the status of the medical profession as we enter the new age of Aquarius.

Realizing the impact of faith healing and that it was becoming recognized as important to the restoration of health, I wanted to know your opinion of the entire health and healing approach today.

Again, to my surprise, I received a tremendous response from both patient and doctor. Patients were rising in protest against their treatment at the hands of doctors. And doctors, many of whom were dear personal friends, were expressing disappointment in their patients, who were reluctant to take any responsibility for their own healing.

Since you informed me overwhelmingly that you wanted more input concerning health and healing, and since you provided me with innumerable tapes and articles to lend credence to your expressions, I have decided to open this book using the relationship of patient-doctor information, as seen from the patients' viewpoint. But remember, even as you read, the doctors' opinions and expressions will follow. Although I share your opinion as it relates to the medical profession in general, I do not join your protest as it relates to the individual doctor. I have many personal friends who are doctors and each is a hard working, wonderful person, totally dedicated to the well-being of his/her patients.

So even though I've begun with what appears to be a scathing indictment against the medical profession, it assuredly does not include the individual doctors with whom I've been associated through the years. Their friendship has been and still is important to me and their dedication to their profession over and above the call of duty has been an inspiration. In the following report, then, responding to your request, and using the information you have forwarded through the years, we'll begin with patient protest as it relates to the search for health and healing.

Patient Dropout

In this chapter let's focus on what is happening on the medical scene — how, as a healer and health consultant, I have witnessed over the years what began as a mild protest against the medical profession, but what has become a rising land-swell of outrage concerning the deterioration of doctor-patient relationship. Not so long ago I was usually sought for prayer help only *after* the patient had exhausted every medication proffered by the physician. The situation seems to have reversed. Healing prayers are now sought first — in a persistent, hopeful effort to avoid the medical approach.

Through past years I met with an occasional request for referral to a holistic type of physician. Now the steady flow has become a stampede. When I suggest that one see a doctor I am immediately rebuffed with either an indignant direct refusal, reluctance, or a request to be referred to a naturopath, acupuncturist-herbalist, osteopath, homeopath, or new age physician familiar with holistic healing. Those reluctant to see an allopathic doctor cite many reasons for their reaction. They complain resentfully of the crowded reception room, the long hours of waiting, assembly line methods of approach, and the downgrading attitude once they do gain the doctor's attention, often for no longer than five or ten minutes. They deeply resent the doctor's failure to guide them toward the nutrition their affliction indicates; to offer any aid whatsoever outside a prescription for drugs; the total rejection of herbs as alternative aids towards healing; and no mention whatever of a program of guidance toward health. Just a quick decision to make a lot of tests, a quicker decision regarding the proper drug to prescribe, and a very large bill to pay upon departure.

"I was just like a number, not a human being. The doctor never even remembered my name. He gave me very little time and handed me mimeographed instructions."

"He listened only halfheartedly, then wrote out a prescription without ever asking about or explaining anything of my problem to me."

"I was always kept waiting many hours. I often had to stand for long stretches in his overcrowded reception room."

"He didn't seem truly attentive, nor did he give me enough time to explain my problem. He just decided upon a test to be made and referred me to another doctor trained to make the test. There wasn't any real time given to determine why I should have the test."

"I was treated like a half-witted child and he made light of my problem."

"He was too impressed with his own importance."

"His office manner was a far cry from a bedside manner — too cold and callous and impersonal."

"He was only available a brief few minutes for consultation, but my bill was outrageous. He was not available, even for phone contact, at any other time."

Obviously ailing humanity is tired of being tired and sick of being sick. And people en masse certainly are sick and tired of the way they are being treated by the medical profession, especially short-term, superficial consultations, the too-hurried diagnosis and the resulting drugs in pills or "shots." Becoming aware that they are often victims of doctor-caused illnesses, many are on a search for a new breed of doctor and they are certainly assuming more responsibility for their health.

Hippocrates, the celebrated Greek physician of 2500 years ago, whose oath the medical profession still swears by, made it quite clear that doctors cannot cure; they can only help the body give nature a chance to heal it. Hippocrates and the ancient physicians always turned to natural methods first, using medication or surgery only as a last resort. (The foremost medication of Hippocrates was honey. For pain he prescribed vinegar and honey.)* Somewhere along the way, probably beginning about 1925, natural methods and folk medicines were eliminated from the doctors' resources. Today, within a few moments of consultation, a prescription for a drug or an injection is given, or the patient is booked for surgery in a hospital, or a number of tests leading toward surgery.

Seldom, if ever, is there a discussion about natural healing, nutrition, naturopathy, acupuncture, homeopathy, exercise, herbs, osteopathy or reflexology. To suggest that diet might be responsible for the problem is often to invoke indifference. The average physician is trained in basic nutrition, but rarely ever integrates nutrition into his or her practice. He usually would not know where to begin to advise the proper change to a natural or purifying diet. If the physician does support a diet it is usually formulated for masses rather than individuals, and consists of processed rather than natural foods. And he can open his medical dictionary, rapidly scan through the thousands of drugs available and pick one that *may* apply to the ailment you *may* have. After determining your ailment, usually you are handed a printed page containing a list of foods everyone with the same disease should eat — usually

*See *The Book of Beginning Again* by Earlyne Chaney, available from Astara, P.O. Box 5003, Upland, CA 91785-5003.

all are processed foods an ailing patient should never eat. Nor does such a dietary consultation help the health-oriented patient who wouldn't dream of eating such foods, even when well. So the money spent on such dietary advice is more than wasted.

In response, patients are deserting conventional doctors by the thousands. Disenchanted by soaring costs, drug abuse and lack of personal interest, they seek a return to illness-prevention and natural methods of healing. They seek a new type of doctor to help them attain this end. They will not refuse to take drugs entirely, but they want longer time given to determine whether or not the drugs are really needed. They fear indiscriminate use of x-rays, which have proven disastrous for so many. But most noticeable of all is the movement toward "I'd-rather-do-it-myself" therapy. And this is the reason I decided to write this book, offering guidelines for those who truly want to help themselves.

I am well aware of the many books available to help you in your struggle to "do-it-yourself." I hope you will find the value of these chapters in their organized plan (or method) of presenting helpful health concepts. They will include exercises, old home remedies, and many other concepts perhaps not readily available in other books. But none of these writings will in any sense be a substitute for a good holistic doctor. One should certainly be consulted in the event of a serious health problem.

This writing will also offer many new drugs which are proving indispensable in the practice of medicine. There is good reason to include these new drugs. You see, discovering the dangers some of their drugs have encountered, medical scientists have broadened their scope for fighting disease. They have gone into the field of the old Indian medicine man, the herbs of the Orientals, the plants of the African witch doctor, the trees of South America and Australia — and have discovered a whole new world of healing. Bringing their discoveries home to their laboratories, they have integrated the herb of the witch doctor, the plant of the medicine man, with their chemicals and drugs and emerged with astonishing potions. Thus we cannot ignore all the amazing new "discoveries" on the medical scene — and I'm happy to share my research with you. Some "drugs" with strange medical names may be powerful herbal remedies long used by the bushmen of the outback.

One of the loudest complaints is that the laboratories of the pharmaceutical houses, using the technique known as "particle synthesis," take the herbs of the witch doctor, add a chemical to give it the right to be called a drug, then patent, process, and market these herbs and plants under strange laboratory code names. The resulting prescriptions usually cost outrageous sums. This is all very splendid, but it obviously removes the herbs from the hands of the herbal doctors and places them in the hands of pharmaceutical companies. Why not grow the herbs and medicinal plants in large fields, process them as herbs, and release them to the public as herbs, clinically proven effective in certain ailments? Is the "chemical push" given so that the pharmaceutical houses may have complete control? Whatever the reason, some of these amazing new medicines will be included so that you may know of them.

Protests from the New Holistic Doctors

A few rare medical practitioners are rising in protest at the incredible state of affairs in the medical profession. Many could be quoted but the words of one of America's foremost doctors, the late personal physician of U. S. Senator Hubert Humphrey, sum up their opinions. Dr. Edgar Berman, author of the book *The Solid Gold Stethoscope* charges that "medicine is going down the drain." He has publicly made a scathing attack against what he finds wrong in the field of medicine. His book clearly states that he feels too many doctors overcharge, perform unnecessary operations, care very little about their patients, over-utilize hospital equipment, turn the office telephone off on weekends and make themselves unavailable. He states that too many doctors are more dedicated to the dollar than to the patient. He has also publicly described the American Medical Association as the "great protector" of doctors and criticized the AMA for failing "to clean out the fraud and incompetence" in the medical profession. He feels 80% of doctors aren't living up to the ethics of their professions.

The late Dr. Robert S. Mendelsohn, former associate professor at the University of Illinois College of Medicine, agreed publicly with Dr. Berman. Many other physicians also concur, but few have made such outspoken accusations.

Dr. Edward Zalta, a California doctor and an executive of Capp Care, the nation's largest Preferred Provider Organization, states that dishonesty is rampant among physicians. He feels that doctors who take advantage of our medical system are driving medical costs far beyond the reach of the average person to pay. He feels such abusers should be indicted and put on trial as criminals. The added costs of such procedures are passed on to everyday working persons in the form of incredibly high insurance premiums. A spokesman for the Aetna Casualty and Life Insurance Company declares that medical costs have become an affront to every American. He blames fraud as the problem. Dr. Sidney Wolfe, of the Public Citizens Health Research Group, maintains that high costs result from widespread unnecessary and inappropriate care. His group estimates that about $180 billion of the $540 billion spent on health care yearly is wasted on unnecessary surgery, hospitalization and other services.

Dr. Halsted R. Holman, professor of medicine at the Stanford University School of Medicine, is another who has raised his voice in protest. A paper he has released charges that some 30-50% of present hospitalizations are medically unnecessary. He accuses physicians of charging outrageous fees. He recognizes that the many people who are now turning to other types of healing and who are realizing effective restoration to health, often fare better than those who seek conventional methodologies. He accuses his colleagues of overusing drugs, and of hospitalizing many people who would be better off treated at home. He believes hospitals are overstocked with tremendously expensive machines which must be paid for through patients being recommended for hospitalization when it is totally unnecessary. He claims that drug overuse produces toxicities which send innumerable people into hospitals.

In other words, the doctor's own methods of healing too often make his patients sick. Dr. Holman thoroughly believes that satisfactory medicine can be approached without using many of the 20 most commonly prescribed drugs. He is convinced that surgery is performed unnecessarily a great share of the time and, finally, he believes customary diagnostic techniques to be totally unsatisfactory. He feels doctors frequently misdiagnose simply through lack of knowledge or lack of sincere concern. The doctors quoted here are to be enthusiastically applauded for their stand. Perhaps they will be joined by many others in time so that the present scandalous condition in the medical field can be remedied.

The Other Side of the Coin

I have dwelt long on the medical "scandal" as it exists today, giving a dark picture concerning the doctor-patient relationship as seen from the patient's viewpoint.

But there are two sides to every coin. What about the doctor's viewpoint — I mean the honest, hard working, sincere, dedicated man or woman who is filled with a true compassionate concern for the welfare of patients — who spends long hours of service proving it? There are many such physicians. Most doctors are extremely busy, harassed, and under pressure. Many conscientiously would like to swerve from giving their patients so many injections, antibiotics, wonder drugs, tranquilizers, and various other pills. Yet they report that when they attempt to persuade the patient to do without the drug therapy and try a healing approach via nutrition and exercise, they meet with stubborn resistance. Patients demand drug therapy. "Come on, doctor, I don't have time for all that stuff. Just give me a shot of something. I have to get back to work."

The doctors grow extremely discouraged and eventually give up the struggle to obtain even partial cooperation or self-help from their patients. Their complaint is that patients seldom want to approach healing through nutritional purification — or any other program except the pill and the needle. Mention of any deviation, such as a change in diet, is met with impatience, disappointment or derision. The public has been brainwashed to believe the doctor's pill or injection will perform the wonders of the "wonder drugs."

I can understand the doctor's frustration. As a healer, I too have met with stubborn reluctance on the part of many healees. . . the ones seeking healing. Experience tells me that many people want help and healing but few really want to be told they must also help themselves. When I mention a change in diet — away from their processed foods, their dead foods, their "delicious" foods — I too often meet with resistance. Traditional beliefs die hard. Even those whose bodies are wracked with pain are often reluctant to make the move back to nature — eating natural foods and taking the steps required for a return to wholeness. Some, because of great suffering, are more than ready to make the change. Others do so through the desire to progress spiritually. But they are rare. These are the truth seekers. These are those who are truly motivated to find the truth — the sufferers and the seekers.

If a patient is told about the possible side effects, he may be considerably more cautious about taking a drug — and the doctor is released from considerable liability if he warns of the dangers and a patient insists on taking the drug anyway. Were this suggestion followed, however, the doctor should be prepared to give his patient help through *other* methods, since many patients wouldn't think of taking a drug once the possible dangers were understood. The doctors should then be familiar with healing through nutrition, herbs, homeopathy, even exercise. Think what a transformation could occur simply by sharing with patients the truth about the drugs prescribed! These fine doctors say they would like to dismiss their present flock of patients and acquire a whole new and different type — those willing to help themselves get well and stay well, along *with* the doctor's help.

Doctors also list among their complaints the patients

who expect him or her to issue a certification of disability when the doctor cannot do so in good conscience. And a surprising number of patients demand regular x-rays when they are totally unnecessary — and expensive lab tests. They insist they need certain dangerous medication, even narcotics. Many insist their "nerves" require some kind of tranquilizer rather than an herb or homeopathic remedy. They read articles about various illnesses and their "cures" through some new drug, and immediately determine their affliction is *that* illness and demand to try the drug. Patients are so drug-oriented and programmed they don't want to try other methods if it requires time and effort on their part. The doctor may realize quite well that if he does not prescribe a get-well-quick drug the patient will march off to another doctor who will.

Doctors complain, too, about seductive patients who hint at sexual favors in exchange for medical services. And patients who misquote their doctor when trying to justify their failure to get well. Strange, too, is a complaint concerning their frustration when a patient doesn't get well after the doctor has done all that can be done — and he/she doesn't know what else to try! This last complaint wasn't against the patient — just a general complaint against the sense of failure when the consequences could be death.

So there you have both sides of the coin. Doctors have their point, too — those who truly realize the potential dangers of healing through drugs. Are you guilty of demanding instant therapy through a pill or an injection? Do you expect the doctor to perform the entire miracle of healing with no help from you? Are you one of those patients your doctor wishes would seek elsewhere for help so he could busy himself with a new type of patient? Next time you see your doctor ask him to share with you information about the drug you're now taking or may be given in the future. If his reaction is negative seek another doctor — and seek until you find a new breed of doctor. Now, since there is a growing group of doctors "turned on" to holistic and new age healing, and since there is a growing mass of people frantically seeking the services of this type of doctor, it is hoped the two can find each other.

The New Age Doctor

Many holistic physicians are now coming to believe that the best possible therapy is a nutritional approach. Discouraged and disillusioned by drug tragedies, they are turning toward vitamin-mineral supplements and nutritional guidance to reestablish wholeness in their patients. Are these splendid physicians — a new species — to be labeled "quacks" simply because they do not follow the orthodox trend? Too often we hear the argument that patients seeking beyond orthodox medicine risk delay in getting proper medical treatment "by going to some quack." But seeking health through nutrition is not quackery — it's letting food be your medicine. Besides, the records clearly show that the majority of patients run the gamut of medical orthodoxy first. Then, physically broken, financially destitute, and mentally disillusioned, they turn in desperation to some "unorthodox" approach.

It could be this approach is simply to seek or offer nutritional guidance. That is much of what my books purport to do. They are intended in no way to diagnose, prescribe, nor "practice medicine." For clarification, let us classify those involved in the world of healing:

1) *A physician or medical doctor:* Is one who has graduated from a school of medicine operating under the medical standards of the country in which it is established. This person has received years of medical training which is supposed to prepare him/her for medical guidance, surgery, general medical practice, or special training in some part of the anatomy. The medical doctor almost always practices allopathic medicine. Allopathy involves medical practice through the use of drugs and chemicals, a few of which are extremely effective in accomplishing a healing, but many very often cause horrendous side effects.

2) *An osteopathic physician*: Usually has the same medical training as the physician, but he adds to his training the knowledge of restoration to physical health through structural balance and manipulation of the body, which he considers to be a vital mechanical organism. He believes that once the body is structurally balanced it may tend to heal itself. Although he, too, occasionally relies upon allopathic medicine he couples it not only with a knowledge of structural and functional balance but, frequently, homeopathy or herbs. The osteopathic doctors usually oppose drugs as remedial agencies. They are opposed to vaccination and serums. They realize some cases require surgical treatment and advocate it as a last resort. They believe many surgical operations are unnecessary and that many operations could be avoided by osteopathic treatment.

3) A *homeopath*: Is one who treats and heals through minute doses of herbs and drugs. This is called homeopathy. He may or may not be a doctor of medicine. He prescribes a remedy that would, in large doses and in a healthy person, produce the same symptoms of which his patient complains — the like-heals-like approach. This is the opposite approach to allopathy. Whereas allopathic

drugs produce effects different from those of the disease treated, the remedies of homeopathy seek to heal by treating the patient with a miniature dose of whatever will produce the same symptoms, arousing inner forces to fight the disease. Thus, in homeopathy, symptoms of old complaints may surface, after which the patient is immunized against the disease. The homeopathic remedy, given in minute doses, immunizes and heals simultaneously. Such a remedy seldom if ever produces dangerous side effects.

4) A *chiropractor*: Is one who has received formal academic training in manipulative techniques to restore wholeness through spinal alignment, pressure on important meridian points, nerve plexuses, heat therapy, ultrasonic therapy, and colonics. He often includes a vitamin-mineral and diet approach to healing.

5) A *naturopath*: Is one who seeks to heal completely through natural methods — chiropracty, homeopathy, nutrition, water therapy, and any kind of approach in tune with nature. The naturopath — who may be a medical physician, a chiropractor, or educated in any medical field — deplores the use of drugs unless they be vitally indicated, and even then he will seek first for a homeopathic or dietary approach.

6) A *nutritionist*: Who also may be trained in a recognized medical field — is one who heals through nutritional guidance. The patient approaching a nutritionist usually already knows what his ailments are and is seeking healing and a restoration to wholeness through nutritional guidance, sometimes with vitamin-mineral therapy added.

7) A *spiritual healer*: Is one who heals through a touch contact, a laying-on-of-hands, or therapy through prayer or affirmative decrees or visualizations. The spiritual healer is sometimes called a psychic healer, psychic surgeon,

faith healer, or practitioner. The learned spiritual healer usually embraces all approaches — the psychic, the practitioner's, the laying-on-of-hands, healing through prayer and, occasionally, nutritional or herbal guidance. If transmitting healing power through the hands is "practicing medicine without a license," then Jesus was the greatest of all offenders. Through his hands, and even his garments, flowed a steady stream of all-powerful healing force, restoring countless individuals to wholeness and regeneration. No one pretends, of course, that healers today can in any way approach his God-powers. But we *can* use the degree of power we *have* developed, remembering always his promise that "as I do, so shall you do also."

For a human to live well on our poor little polluted planet these days, it should be obvious that no single therapy is complete within itself, and we have need of every approach to healing.

For many years chiropractors, homeopaths, naturopaths, nutritionists and faith healers came under attack from medical physicians. But the picture is rapidly changing as more and more physicians take a second look at drug therapy. And they are rapidly recognizing the faith healer as a positive approach to healing. And many brave doctors, such as those quoted, are speaking out against practices in their own field of allopathic medicine.

Many fault the American Medical Association, saying it has established a powerful lobby in Congress and uses its staggering influence through lawsuits, threats, and other tactics to prevent others from approaching new methods and new techniques of healing. The AMA finally was ordered by a court to send letters to all 270,000 members of the AMA, saying doctors can now confer with or recommend chiropractors if they think it is in the best interest of their patients. And some now have a chiropractor as a part of their clinical staff. We all realize there are "quacks" and charlatans in the field of health and healing, but there are also thousands upon thousands of sincere, well-trained osteopaths, homeopaths, chiropractors, naturopaths, healers and nutritionists equally qualified to restore health. Just as there are charlatans among the nonmedical practitioners, so are there many among the medical physicians.

Certainly we all know we have need of modern medicine, surgery when needed, and a limited use of drug therapy. But many are thoroughly convinced that an effective, holistic approach to healing today should include homeopathy, osteopathy, chiropracty, naturopathy, nutrition and spiritual or faith healing. God, our Creator, has given us a most marvelous sensitive instrument which we call "*the body*." In His incomparable wisdom He created every part to function smoothly and harmoniously with all the other parts. In the brain He built an incredible cosmic television-computer mechanism, a system of vision with which to behold the wonders of His planet. He added the potential to "see" higher realms, higher worlds. He gave a hearing mechanism with which to catch the sounds of His physical world. And He added the potential to tune in, under proper circumstances, and listen to the Sound Current of the spheres. He gave a voice with which to communicate with others and, in its highest potential, He gave it power to chant His name.

If millions of these "bodies" He designed for us are now out of harmony it is not because God did not know how to construct them. It is simply that we, in our human ignorance, have poisoned and polluted these incredibly intricate instruments and have turned a marvelous walking miracle into a broken and beaten remnant of what might have been. Mother Nature — who helped create this marvelous instrument — does not tolerate the breaking of her laws. And when we, her children, break them, she allows us to pay the penalty. One of our greatest "sins" against these bodies is to assume that the humans calling themselves "doctors" are miniature gods who are all-wise, who know all the answers to our physical problems. We have placed in their hands our physical destinies and many have exploited and misunderstood our bodies to the fullest extent.

The first basic complaint is that, in our medical training systems, the student doctor is taught nothing about natural methods of healing. He is only taught drug therapy, drug therapy, drug therapy — and surgery. He is not taught to analyze the patient as a human being, with a body, a mind and spirit. He is only taught that certain drugs should be given once a diagnosis has been established. The training fails to include adequate studies concerning nutrition, herbs and other holistic approaches, and their effect on the health and healing of the body. Certainly that man or woman who progresses through four years of college, four years of medical school, a period of internship, then special training to become a specialist, is to be applauded. Such lengthy study requires considerable perseverance and dedication.

The principal fault of the entire system lies in the fact that, with all that training, the student doctor is not given adequate knowledge concerning alternative methodologies and their effect upon our health and well-being. He or she is not enlightened concerning the effect of the additives in our food upon the anatomy, for example. What is happening is: 1. Very often the diagnosis is incorrect.

2. The drug prescribed for the ailment often makes the patient more ill than the original complaint.

Yet we are all aware of the millions of dollars poured into medical research and pleas for more — millions for cancer, heart, arthritis, diabetes, Parkinson's disease, emphysema, cerebral palsy, mental illness, muscular dystrophy, multiple sclerosis, epilepsy, and on and on. What is happening to our millions? More important, what is happening to the patients?

Those in America's medical establishment (and others around the world, too) use many drugs which are most destructive to the human anatomy. On the other hand, they often are forbidden to use those which for years have proven excellent in other countries — and even in our own country, in some cases. There have been several cancer "cures" discovered by respected medical researchers, but these "cures" have been called fraudulent, and those fostering them have been called "quacks," even though physicians involved in these discoveries were highly respected medical researchers.

The Trapped Doctor — When hospitals invest massive sums in new types of equipment, the doctors on the staff are expected to keep the hospital beds filled in order for the hospital to pay the vast expenses. They are also expected to refer numerous patients for treatment with the equipment so the fees will enable the hospital to pay for it. Thus, the unsuspecting patient gets caught up in a vicious cycle. He often becomes simply the means whereby the doctor and the hospital keep functioning. Whether surgery is needed or not, the patient is often scheduled for it. The doctor is keenly aware that, being part of a hospital staff, he is expected to provide the hospital with his quota of patients, enabling the hospital to meet its overhead and pay for the laboratory equipment. If enough patients were simply placed on the proper diets and given herbal or natural remedies, many hospitals would no longer be overcrowded.

Iatrogenic Ailments — Iatrogenic ailments are those which a patient develops because of drugs given him by his physician — drugs which were meant to heal a malady, but which create a disease worse than the one they were intended to cure. For instance, penicillin: many thousands can take it safely; many more thousands are allergic to the point of death. The same is true of most other "wonder drugs." The public is becoming very aware that antibiotics and wonder drugs should be carefully considered before introducing them into the human system.

Drug Overkill — Dr. Alexander Schmidt, retired commissioner of the Food and Drug Administration, states that millions of unsuspecting patients face serious injury or death because reckless physicians are overprescribing potent drugs.

"This has become a major national problem with some drugs — especially mood-altering drugs, hormones, vitamins, minerals and, to a lesser degree, antibiotics. I'm appalled with testimony at several Congressional hearings where repeatedly it is demonstrated that physicians overprescribed and misused drugs. The testimony has documented the disastrous effects of such misprescribing which has sometimes caused needless injury or death."

A paper describing the possible side effects of every drug prescribed should be given to each patient. A patient has the right to know the potential side effects he or she may experience before allowing a potentially harmful substance to enter the body. The doctor is well aware of the possible side effects — they are fully described in his medical dictionary. Yet for some reason doctors rarely take time to warn a patient, or they feel it is not wise to "suggest" to the patient that he/she may have adverse reactions. Thus when a drug is prescribed, you should insist on being told its possible side effects. Ask what adverse reaction may be expected so that, if a reaction occurs, you know quite well it was caused by the drug.

Ghost Surgery — Do you know what is meant by "ghost surgery?" It means that if you are planning to submit to surgery and you believe a certain doctor, an expert, is going to perform the operation, you may be totally misguided. In many hospitals today your private surgeon does not perform the operation. An inexperienced resident doctor may do so with the surgeon looking on and instructing him. Unfortunately, many times the inexperienced resident performs the operation when the private doctor is not even present, or he may leave before it is complete. *"It happens in millions of cases,"* said E. Donald Chappero, dean of the New York Law School and adjunct professor of Preventive Medicine at New York University Medical School. *"Many patients have been injured for life when an inexperienced resident surgeon performed an operation he was not qualified to perform."* So, if you face an operation in the future make very sure who will do the actual surgery.

Blood Transfusion — If you are scheduled for surgery you have a right to ask that you not be given a blood transfusion unless it is a matter of life and death. Jehovah's Witnesses refuse blood transfusions because of their religious beliefs, nor can they be compelled to submit to a transfusion. A group at the Texas Heart Institute in Houston have released a report that some blood vessel surgery is now accomplished on Jehovah's Witness patients without the need for transfusion. All cut blood vessels are rapidly and meticulously clamped to prevent excessive bleeding, and blood loss is immediately replaced with a solution of salt, carbohydrate, potassium and calcium during and after the operation to keep the circulation stable. Dr. C. Wilson Simmons, Jr., states: "*Vascular surgery is routinely performed in this hospital without blood transfusion unless specifically indicated. Blood is used cautiously during and after operations and patients who refuse to accept blood can usually undergo major operations without a prohibitive risk and enjoy favorable post-operative results.*"

Hospital records indicate that a great share of people who are given blood transfusions suffer reactions such as jaundice and hepatitis. Frequently death is the result, or many months of extreme discomfort when a blood transfusion may not have been at all necessary. With AIDS so prevalent doctors are now cautious about transfusions. It is well to find a friend or relative prior to surgery to offer blood. Or even report to the hospital before surgery to give your own blood to be used, if necessary, during surgery.

The Future

When I think of the medical profession I feel both glad and sad. Sad because for so many years many doctors have viewed a patient not as a whole person, but as a certain disease which needed treating. Often they have treated the symptoms, not the *cause* of the disease. Many were sadly ignorant concerning nutrition and all the laws of health and regeneration.

Glad because *now* we are entering a time when holistic healing is coming to the fore — which is to say that doctors are beginning to realize man is more than body. He is a spirit with a soul, a mind and a body, all of which need consideration in a regeneration and healing program. As the holistic healing program advances — healing for the whole person, not just for the body and the disease — we shall begin to see more and more doctors turning toward new age medicine — natural diet, yoga, deep breathing and breath control, biofeedback, acupressure, acupuncture, herbs, reflexology, kinesiology, and many methods the old naturopaths advocated years ago. Many of us, searching out the proper doctor, have previously searched in vain for one trained to heal the whole person. They are becoming easier to find and, as the movement spreads, perhaps we shall see the day when the holistic physician will be the rule instead of the unusual.

Presently physicians are required to refer constantly to the chemical medicines listed in the Physician's Desk Reference. The AMA stipulates that he can use no other chemicals or drugs. To do so means risking his license as a physician. The Federal Drug Administration controls the listing of the drugs and chemicals in the reference book. Every listing must be approved by the Federal Drug Administration. Thus the physicians are working directly under the control of the FDA — which, in turn, seems to operate under the control of the giant drug industries, the manufacturers of all the drugs now flooding the medical scene. So the allopathic is, again, the "trapped" doctor. If he deviates too far from the beaten path, he/she may find themselves the beaten. Somehow, some way the medical scene must change. But it will take time and courage.

The National Health Federation, P. O. Box 688, Monrovia, CA 91016, was organized to oppose traditional tactics of the American Medical Association and to seek freedom of choice for patients who desire to seek health and healing through holistic, unconventional and natural methods. It is the consensus of a great mass of people that the AMA has no right to prevent an individual from receiving the treatment he desires, nor has it the right to prevent a fellow doctor from issuing a quality-controlled medication he may truly feel would be beneficial to his patient. Write for membership information if you wish.

Chapter Two

The "Why" Chapter

Let's begin this chapter as an extension of the last one — but with a few "whys" that urgently require answers. Our first "why" takes the form of a persistent question as to *why* our government does not establish research laboratories to determine the effect of chemicals and preservatives in our food in relation to our national health? Why not address the question of whether or not much of our diseases and complaints can ultimately be traced to bad nutrition? Why all the billions spent on *cures* rather than natural prevention? — billions for cancer research, multiple sclerosis, Parkinson's, heart, diabetes, and on and on — and no real focus on the *cause* behind these disasters?

Let's just say that the government *did* establish these nutrition-herbal research centers and released their reports that nutrition and herbal therapy were indeed turning around the dismal health scene in America. Let's say the doctors stopped giving most of their questionable drugs and started learning how to guide patients toward health via natural remedies — nutrition, herbs, exercise, massage and meditation. What, then, would become of all the multimillion dollar pharmaceutical industries involved in producing high-powered drugs? And all those chemical plants that chemicalize our food? What would become of the giant junk food industries? Where, suddenly, their massive profits? And what if our U. S. Department of Agriculture asked our food farmers to grow food organically rather than with chemicals? Would our major illnesses decrease? — the heart problem? Cancer?

Assuredly, illness *is* big business — cancer the most lucrative of all. Let's just consider cancer a moment — which leads us to our second "why." Why does not medical science include the role of nutrition or herbs in a cancer cure or prevention? The treatment always accorded those who discover a possible cancer cure is deplorable. They have their medical license removed to prevent them from further research or treatment of patients. Their careers and reputations are ruined. Why does the AMA seem so determined to prevent new possible cancer cures?

What of all those cancer cures we heard about in years gone by — cures discovered by highly respected medical scientists — William Koch, Ivy, Hoxsey, Drones-Lazenby, the Krebiazon team? Information abounds concerning a cancer cure through diet, herbs and proper exercise. Jason Winters, whose cancer first went into remission through Laetrile, a natural remedy made from apricot kernels, and then later through herbs, offers his herbal formula now for sale in most health stores. Yet billions are still spent seeking a cure. Why will they never turn the full scope of research upon prevention? — upon herbs, upon the negative effect of diet — the effect of additives on the body — additives and cancer in laboratory tests? *Why?* Hanna Kroeger, a tiny German woman known nationally for her natural herbal and homeopathic remedies, has submitted the following chart for publication in this book, concerning additives in our food:

Bottom Line: Food Additives

"The subject of chemical food additives is not a new one in the health field. Initially, these preservatives, colorings and other chemicals were thought to be the best thing that ever happened to the food business. These additives prolong shelf-life, maintain colors and preserve good flavor. The Bottom Line, however, is that although these chemicals reduced waste and increased sales, they simply did not know the long-term consequences of pouring these chemicals into our bodies. Now it seems everyone has some idea of how harmful these chemicals are, but still they remain a major part of the processed food industry and our diet. The following chart will shed some light on the subject of food additives so that through our awareness of these chemicals we can further prevent their threat to our good health.

Additive	Chemical Uses	Health Risks
MSG (Monosodium Glutamate — salt substitute)	Flavor enhancer used in canned and frozen foods, prepared meats, pickles, soups, candy, baked goods, mayonnaise, Accent (100% MSG) and in many Chinese foods.	Affects nerve endings; can cause dizziness, numbness, headaches and other symptoms.

Additive	Chemical Uses	Health Risks
Yellow dye #5	Yellow coloring found in beverages, candy cereals, ice cream, baked goods, snack foods, also in prescription drugs, pain relievers and antihistamines.	Can cause allergic reactions, including wheezing, asthmatic symptoms and hives.
BHA (Butylated Hydroxyanisole)	Prevents fats and oils from turning rancid in shortenings, potato chips, cereals, desserts, pudding, candy and bakery products.	Can cause allergic reactions.
BHT(Butylated Hydroxytoluene)	Prevents fats and oils from turning rancid in potato flakes, enriched rice, shortenings containing animal fats, frozen pork sausage and freeze dried meats.	Can cause allergic reactions. Tests produced chemical changes in brains of test animal offspring.
Glycerides	Emulsifying and defoaming agent found in bakery products, ice cream, ice milk, lard, chewing gum, shortening, margarine, sweet chocolate and whipped toppings.	Suspected of causing reproductive problems and malformations.

Additive	Chemical Uses	Health Risks
Red Dye #2 Blue Dye #1	Coloring found in soft drinks, desserts, candies, cereals, bakery products and cherries.	Produced tumors in test animals. Can cause allergic reactions.
Nitrites and Nitrates (Potassium and Sodium)	Used as a color fixative in cured meats, meat spreads, pickling, brine smoked ham, ground meat, poultry, smoked fish and some meat tenderizers.	Combines with other substances to produce cancerous agents called nitrosamines and nitrosamides. May reduce flow of oxygen to the brain and heart.
Sulphur Dioxide	Prevents foods from spoiling and/or fermenting; used in dried fruits like raisins and prunes, used in wines, corn syrup, dehydrated potatoes, soups and condiments.	Tends to deplete the body's supply of vitamin A. Inhalation can cause respiratory irritation."

Continuing our *whys* — if Red Dye #2 and Blue #1 produced tumors in test animals, why is it still allowed in soft drinks, desserts (ice cream), candies, cherries, bakery products, etc.? Wouldn't it also produce tumors in people? If Yellow Dye #5 causes asthmatic symptoms, why isn't it printed on labels of prescription drugs, pain relievers and antihistamines? — just as the Surgeon General issues a warning on cigarettes? Think of all those millions suffering from asthma who are innocent victims of such a dye in many of their foods to which they are allergic. And monosodium glutamate! — in *so* many foods! Almost all frozen dinners contain it. Its effect is so dreadful, many Chinese restaurants now post a huge sign on their windows *We do not use* MSG, so that their customers may be informed. MSG can trigger a headache so devastating no pain reliever can ease it. I know — I'm a victim who discovered its effect. But what of all those millions who eat frozen dinners, weight control dinners, pastas, etc., who don't read labels and who wonder why they have migraine headaches! Nitrites and nitrates are so dangerous they should *never* be in our foods, even with a warning on the label — yet I'm told they are even used in canned baby foods.

Our next "why" involves the x-ray. Did you know that an overdose of x-ray causes cancer? Did you know that radiation under certain conditions can cause hereditary defects — sterility, deformed bodies, susceptibility to mental diseases? Did you know that x-ray is cumulative, building up in your system over the years? Did you know that every x-ray to which you submit adds to the radioactivity which your body has already accumulated? How many children now dying of leukemia were treated in earlier childhood with extensive x-rays — or exposed while still in the womb by mother's x-rays?

Americans have never been properly educated concerning the deadly form of delayed action of x-rays on their physical system. You enter a dentist's office every few months and often submit to a routine x-ray oral examination. It doesn't hurt to have an x-ray so we seldom pause to protest these "routine" procedures.

Medical and dental x-rays are creating troubles for generations yet unborn and many of us already born are walking laboratories of x-ray overexposure. Did you know you get at least five roentgen units from one dental x-ray? And did you know that a fraction of that dental x-ray "spills over" — strays — into the reproductive organs? All of us are constantly exposed to some background radiation from outer space, from the gram of radium that exists in a square mile of the earth's soil. The body is built to repair minor radiation damage continuously. Damaged tissues even have a chance to recover from this gradual absorption — but our bodies are no match for our machines. Your doctor is not altogether to blame. If he fails to perform an x-ray when an x-ray may be indicated, he may be legally liable for malpractice. But any time x-ray can be sensibly avoided, do so. For anything less than cancer, x-ray should be used with extreme caution. Don't you be one of the steady stream of patients sent in for an x-ray exposure simply as a routine practice.

Having warned at length concerning x-ray overkill, it is only fitting that I offer suggestions about combating the effect of radiation in the body — since there seems to be no alternative in some cases of illness or physical examinations. Some holistic researchers insist that, following x-rays, one should take a full tub bath to which has been added two cups (one pound) of Epsom salts and two cups (one pound) of baking soda. Or salt from a health store (not iodized) may be used. Soak for twenty minutes and repeat the tub soak twice a week for a month. Others suggest massive dosages of Superoxide Dismutase (SOD). Eight tablets should be taken in the morning for two days prior, and eight in the morning for two days following x-rays. The ordinary tablet contains 125 mcg. (micromilligrams), but to be effective against radiation the tablets should contain more massive units. Consult your holistic physician. Others prescribe a homeopathic remedy called *Radium Brom 30X*, taken daily four days prior to x-rays. You may wish to use all three methodologies since none are harmful.

Tranquilizers Can Kill You

Why the indiscriminate use of billions of tranquilizing tablets? The growing use of "happiness" pills has reached the danger point, both for individuals and the nation. Millions are unwitting victims of a dangerous practice. Many prominent physicians are expressing deep concern over the growing tendency to seek tranquilizers as buffers against the stresses and strains of modern living.

Tranquilizers containing the drug *Meprobamate* can greatly increase the intoxicating effects of alcoholic beverages. Physicians have been urged to warn patients who are taking Meprobamate, especially if they are likely to operate moving vehicles or other complex machinery. Among the drugs that contain Meprobamate are *Milltown*, *Equinil*, *Meprospan*, and *Meprotabs*. They are prescribed for stress and insomnia among other ills. Researchers are looking for a combined effect of Meprobamate and alcohol on performance. Concerning one test, they wrote that they were "frankly not prepared for the extent of the effects."

If you do not take tranquilizers you may naturally assume that such a problem does not concern you. Unfortunately, it does. Many people drink socially and then drive. Most do not drink to excess. But if they also take tranquilizers, there is danger. Any widely used drug which greatly increases the effect of alcohol is a distinct menace to users and nonusers alike. Here we have a possible explanation of the appalling increase of death on the highways. You may be a perfectly safe driver, obeying all the rules of the road, but if another driver's reactions are impaired by a combination of tranquilizers and alcohol you may be his innocent victim. And the chances of your becoming involved in such an accident are steadily increasing. The effects of tranquilizers are so pronounced that the Armed Services are reported to require that any military pilot refrain from flying at the controls of jet aircraft for at least two months after taking such drugs.

Why not herbs as an alternative? — especially for insomnia. Many osteopaths, medical doctors and chiropractors suggest *Good Night Herb* capsules, or *Silent Night, Calms Forte*, *Kalm Caps*, *Relax-Plex*, and homeopathic remedies, all available at health stores. Most of these products produce drowsiness, because they contain herbal ingredients renowned for relaxation and insomnia, such as Passaflora, Henbane, Kali Phosphoricum, Hops, Chamomile, Valerian Root and Skullcap. None of these herbal remedies are addictive.

****

Throughout this book I'll be listing products or companies where products may be obtained. To provide an easy to find guide, I'll list the addresses of these companies and their products in the last chapter. So when, in the text, I say *address elsewhere*, it means you should seek the address in the last chapter.

Chapter Three

Are We Smarter Than God?

It all started with Napoleon who, early in the 19th century, offered a reward to anyone who could devise a method of food preservation to facilitate feeding his vast armies which were always on the march. Responding to this challenge a chemist, after years of experimenting, discovered how to preserve cooked food in glass jars. But it was not until 1810, just prior to the Civil War, that the steel, tin-coated can was introduced by Englishman Peter Duran, which immediately posed a problem. How to open the can! Directions on the label instructed the use of chisel and hammer — tapping the chisel with a hammer as the can was rotated slowly. Thus were the cans opened until 1867, when the can opener was invented.

A serious problem soon developed. Canned foods stored for long periods resulted in swollen, puffed cans because the food inside had spoiled. The condition was caused by a bacterial poison called "botulism." This toxin spread throughout the canned food. The toxin caused many deaths, since no known antidote or treatment was available. The infant canning industry suffered a serious setback. For many years the public avoided commercially canned goods, fearing the deadly toxins. Housewives, however, began to realize they could safely can their garden vegetables at home for one season and then dispose of the remainder to their chickens.

But the day of home canning for necessity is long since passé. Millions of housewives now file through the checkout counters of supermarkets carting home fruits, vegetables, and other produce synthetically processed with just about every known chemical preservative. Although these chemicals prevent spoiling by bacteria that produces botulism in canned goods, the "overkill" use of such preservatives has deadly side effects. We are now faced with the food-additive problem, which involves the use of innumerable synthetically derived chemicals. One of the first preservatives was sodium benzoate, which enabled the food processors, distributors and speculators to keep warehouses full of canned food for indefinite periods. With the passing years the chemical food industry added a growing list of new preservatives derived from the sodium radical combined with coal tar derivatives. In addition, a formidable array of cheap, synthetically produced food colors and flavors were also added.

These petrochemicals constitute a vast segment of American industry. They are used by nearly all food processors, who maintain a lobby in Congress and wield powerful pressure to prevent investigation into their products. It should be well known by every investigative congressional body and the FDA that it has been thoroughly established beyond the shadow of doubt that coal tar causes cancer. In every possible laboratory test this fact has been proven over and over. Yet today there are well over one thousand coal tar derivatives used in our food, drinks and medicines — tons of questionable substances foisted upon an unsuspecting public. Life on Earth can assuredly be hazardous to your health — especially eating.

Conscientious doctors occasionally release a report on the harmful effects of chemicals and dyes. They frankly state that laboratory experiments prove they cause cancer. Many products containing artificial coal tar dye are renowned for starting cancer in laboratory animals. Now do you understand why we urge you not to eat processed, chemicalized food? When even our own Food and Drug Administration refuses to ban such dangerous chemical food additives and dyes who can we look to for protection? It would seem they are far more interested in protecting the interests of the chemical companies who manufacture the dyes and chemicals than they are in the safety of the public. All we can do is urge you to avoid these processed foods. The unsuspecting public can hardly tell the difference between that which nature made and that which the chemical companies make — and actually seem not to care. Perhaps it's because the general public is not aware of the poisonous danger in processed products.

Processed foods include fruits, vegetables, *canned pressed meats*, candy, cookies, pies, cakes, soft drinks such as Coca Cola, potato chips, roasted and salted nuts, white flour, white sugar, white salt, coffee cake, pastries, bread made with white flour, sugar-coated cereals, ice cream, instant breakfasts, instant coffee, doughnuts, hot dogs, bologna, TV dinners, Jell-o, gelatins, cake icing, jams, jellies, margarine, frozen dinners, weight reducing dinners, pastas.

About processing foods, Robert S. Harris, Ph.D., of the Department of Nutrition and Food Science at the Massachusetts Institute of Technology, says that by the time processed foods reach you, "they may have been shipped and stored, trimmed, blanched, frozen, canned, condensed, dehydrated, pasteurized, sterilized, smoked, cured, milled, roasted, cooked, toasted, or puffed. What's left of their composition after any combination of those tortures is then liable to be further stolen by heat, light, oxygen, oxylates, antivitamins, acidity, alkalinity, metal catalysts, enzymes, and irradiation. But that is only the beginning of the abuse of natural foods. To this weird substance agricultural science dares to call food, is added nitrates, nitrites, preservatives, all manner of chemicals and dyes."

Scientific magazines, and even our daily newspapers, often report prophecies of our bright future, all glittering and trouble-free. Somehow, we shall only need to push a button and get a complete chemicalized meal from a coded card. That is supposed to be advanced living — no one will have to worry about cooking any more, the processed food manufacturers will do it all for us. And all the while we get sicker and sicker.

These prophetic articles never mention the plight of the average person who sees his savings dwindle in the payment of doctor and hospital bills, often to no avail. These reports never mention the sterility affecting many millions of Americans, the cancer deaths, the millions of arthritis victims, the sudden death from heart failure, and the slow, painful agony of the chronic sufferer. Nor do they enlighten us concerning experiments conducted on laboratory rats and mice, fed on minute percentages of chemicals now added to our daily food — experiments that brought the animals to their deaths. This is not to belittle the many miracles medical science produces. But it should also automatically report to the public the results of experiments on chemicals in human nutrition.

There can be little doubt that the swing toward holistic medicine — and somewhat of a return to natural healing — is far overdue. It's not that the principles are actually new, it's just that perhaps we are beginning to understand the incredible damage the pharmaceutical houses, the food industries, and the chemical manufacturers have done to America in their greed for prosperity — their own.

Cancer and Food Additives

Medical researchers declare cancer to be a great mystery. Billions have been spent on medical research to discover a cure but, again, very little to find the cause. As a matter of fact, it requires no monetary expenditure whatsoever. It's very simple. Why need all those billions be spent on a cure when the main source and cause points toward diet: the additives, the coal tar, the preservatives, the dye, the chemicals? The medical profession and the entire populace is now well aware that the diet is very much involved in heart problems, and certainly in diabetes. If diet is involved in any one disease, isn't it reasonable to connect diet with other diseases? Why not cancer? At the moment the solution seems to rest only in the hands of the individual who, becoming aware, begins to instigate a diet change — first purchasing organically grown vegetables when available, then reducing meat consumption.

The outcry against "junk food" in general has been echoed by top nutritionists, and at the head of their list are cola-flavored drinks. Dr. Emory Thurston, president of the Institute of Nutritional Research, states: "All soft drinks are terrible because of the sugar they contain. But cola-flavored ones are worse still because they also contain caffeine in a far more potent form than the caffeine in coffee or tea."

Other foods to be avoided, according to top nutritional experts, are:

1) "Fruit drinks" because they are 90% water, sugar and chemicals — very little fruit at all.

2) Heavily salted snack foods (refined white salt) which increase water retention, leading to high blood pressure — roasted salted nuts, crackers, pressed meats, pretzels, chips, etc.

3) Hydrogenated fats, such as margarine and solid shortening.

4) Commercially frozen desserts and ice cream, which are not really food, but thinly disguised "chemical feasts." Many brands are made of chemical substitutes and other dangerous additives.

5) Imitation foods, such as dairy substitutes and instant breakfasts, imitation "eggs" — all filled with chemicals and dangerous additives, and offering little nutrition.

The food industries claim that using the additives makes it possible for them to supply the housewife with cheaper packaged food and that, without their preservatives, food costs would rise sharply because of spoilage and other factors. Of course it is recognized that some preservative additive is necessary to protect packaged foods. But surely not an array as is now added. How many millions may have died with heart attacks, cancer, arteriosclerosis, multiple sclerosis and other horrendous diseases directly due to these chemical additives?

No nation on earth chemicalizes its food as America does, and no nation on earth has the modern degenerative diseases with which Americans suffer. More and more processed food packages appear on the supermarket shelves daily, containing flavorings, preservatives, chemical dyes, emulsifiers, monosodium glutamate, extenders, thickeners, sweeteners, hydrogenators, anti-caking agents, inhibitors, artificial coloring, and on and on. The food additive business continues to thrive by leaps and bounds, far beyond the power of the FDA to cope with the problem. And Congress shows little interest or inclination to tackle the giant food industry, which grows richer and richer while the health of Americans grows constantly poorer.

The FDA, whose chief function is to see that the public obtains pure food, is constantly harassed by groups who represent food manufacturers seeking cheaper methods of production which will increase profits and meet competition. The farm community itself has faced many problems since the tremendous migration of people from the farms to the cities. The majority of farmers also buy their food from the supermarket, themselves specializing in a single product such as cotton, wheat, corn, or other staple commodity.

While this tremendous evolution of processed foods has been taking place over the years, the American public has accepted it with inertia, seeming unaware of being slowly poisoned. It's a matter of having faith — faith in one's government, faith in one's governmental agencies — faith that the Food and Drug Administration would perform the job intended, never dreaming that individuals inside the agency itself would succumb to the pressure of the food manufacturers and turn their backs upon the potential danger to the very people they are supposed to protect.

A Strange New "Meat" for America

Did you know that some countries — especially Scandinavian countries — forbid the sale of any meat for human consumption obtained from animals raised on farms in the United States? An explanatory report stated that "the meat they eat in the U.S.A. is fit for pigs." The article deplored the advanced technology which makes possible artificial fattening of cattle, through tranquilizers which increase their appetite, and massive use of sex hormones. They specifically focused on hot dogs with triturated bones and fats. What these Scandinavian countries are saying is that they are now alerted to the corporate desire for more profits in our country by fattening cattle and hogs faster and faster through artificial means so that they may be heavier and available for market sooner.

All of us are very proud of the "know how" in America in accomplishing great things — but not in the meat industry. Such "industrial and technological advances" enabled the meat industry to add 20% of pulverized bones and fat to their hot dogs, and other indescribable meat by-products to their sausages, hamburgers, and all processed meats, both canned and cured. With nature's methods alone it requires three to four years for cattle to be able to provide beef. But by using hormones to produce artificial fat and tranquilizers to increase appetite, beef can be on the American dinner table between one and one-and-a-half years. Even when the cattle grazes on "natural" pasture they eat pesticides and chemical fertilizers which leave their residue in the meat of the animal. In addition, on many commercial farms animals are persuaded to eat constantly by means of artificial lights which burn around the clock, creating in the beasts the false notion of endless day.

One of the mixtures used to fatten the animals is of urea and carbohydrates added to a high protein diet. Discovering that the animal required vitamin A to fatten quickly, synthetic vitamin A is now given, not to improve the meat but only to fatten it.

Could it be that eating meat and poultry laced with synthetic hormones, antibiotics, etc. is the main reason Americans are habitually overweight? If the additives will fatten animals for marketing, couldn't they also fatten humans who eat the flesh containing the hormones and the additives?

Antibiotics are used to make the fat in the meat appear white and hard, instead of the normal look of yellowish and soft. The harm comes because the fat produced by the antibiotics contains great quantities of cholesterol — the very item against which medics warn Americans. The antibiotic is called *nitrite*, which has caused innumerable poisonings among infants and younger children. It was once and may still be used very freely in baby food. Not only that, but when the nitrite combines with other chemical products it is often turned into carcinogenic — or cancer-producing — substances. Finally, just prior to the day the animal is to be sold on the market, it is injected with chemical products to make the animal retain the liquid which normal biological processes would eliminate, but which cause them to weigh more when being sold. So, meat-eaters, take note. Use processed foods and meat at your own risk. You may not be eating meat at all, but only a meat product injected with innumerable chemicals, hormones, antibiotics, and artificial flavoring.

One antibiotic used in the feed of pigs and cows to cut down on a variety of diseases among livestock, as well as speeding the growth of the animals, is sulfamethazine. In 1975, the Department of Agriculture and the FDA discovered that 15% of all pork sold in the United States contained residues of sulfamethazine that exceeded the federal safety limits. The FDA, after 14 years of study, is now moving to ban its use altogether since their studies show a clear relationship to its use and cancerous tumors of the thyroid glands of mice.

In the 1920s cancer among children was a rarity. Today some form of cancer in children and babies at birth is a frequent occurrence. One could continue to itemize and tabulate the dreary statistics covering allergic diseases, nervous disorders, degenerative heart diseases, arteriosclerosis, arthritis, epilepsy, and many other gloomy categories of human woes and ailments, but it simply leads to the obvious conclusion that well over half of our nation is afflicted with some type of chronic disease. Something must be drastically wrong. We healthians — healers and holistic physicians — are convinced that the contaminatives, additives and toxic chemical compounds taken into the human body through food and drink are, in large measure, responsible for the deplorable deterioration of our national health.

Americans appear to be the most overfed nation on earth but the most undernourished. There are almost a thousand different toxic chemical compounds used in our foods. How could we possibly fail to realize that these chemicals constitute a calculated risk to human health, even life itself? The human body is built to utilize only natural foods as nourishment. Chemicals are not natural food elements and, taken into the body, can only produce harmful results.

Many American housewives, wheeling their carts innocently around the supermarket, are becoming more aware that there must be a connection between the incidence of degenerative diseases, such as cancer and heart disease, and the phenomenal increase in the total amount of chemical compounds added to our foods — there must exist a causal connection. The invariable concurrence of disease and body contamination by the consumption of toxic chemicals must be more than coincidental. And many millions are now seeking fresh vegetables and fruits. They are eating less flesh food and concentrating on soy products, grains, dairy proteins, nuts and legumes for protein.

What you must never forget is that these chemical compounds are cumulative in the cells and tissues of the body. Not only that, they often cause a reaction with natural body chemicals since the body itself is a natural chemical plant. God, the greatest of all alchemists, made the body a chemical producer of insulin, bile, hydrochloric acid, and innumerable others. Man's synthetically derived chemicals simply do not harmonize with God's natural chemicals. With such a chemicalized diet the body's natural chemical balance is disrupted and thrown out of harmony, inevitably resulting in some type of illness. The reports concerning the overall picture of American health records are not only shocking, they are appalling. Certainly, if no organized universal action is taken, at least we, as individuals, can look to our own reevaluation. If the health of America is slowly deteriorating, need we light seekers be among the victimized masses?

Chapter Four

The Colon: Its Secret of Life and Death

Time was when, given a hundred people, fifty would be suffering from some kind of colon or intestinal distress, either through constipation, diarrhea, or both. Now, given a hundred people, almost one hundred will be experiencing some form of intestinal problem — be it constipation, diarrhea, lack of digestive enzymes, diverticulitis, ulcers, and on and on.

Nothing is more precious to life than good health. The wealthiest person in the world is brought low when health fails. Illness is an effect, and behind every effect is a cause. One of the prolific causes of ill health is constipation. A large percentage of the ills from which we suffer, particularly a majority of the headaches, skin eruptions, and disorders arising from impure blood, are largely the result of toxic poisons due to constipation. A sluggish colon, impacted with fermenting and partly digested food, is the underlying cause of most physical problems. The foul toxins of such a colon are reabsorbed by the general processes of the body's chemistry, entering every cell, tissue and muscle, and slowly poisoning the entire body.

When one eats cooked food saturated with chemicals, dyes, additives, it acts as foreign substance in the colon. The body, protecting the system against invading foreign matter, automatically produces mucus. When such food is eaten day after day, year after year, the colon becomes a canal of solidified mucus. The majority seek to relieve the congestion with pills and other laxatives, which is not a sensible approach. When the stomach and intestinal tract are unable to perform their natural function, ill health is inevitable. Autointoxication is a natural result. A vicious cycle of action and reaction begins. The majority of humankind is self-intoxicated by fermenting inner poisons. The liver, kidneys and heart are overworked. You begin to decline in energy. Aches and pains develop, and you grow old while you still should be fresh and young. Age is not a matter of years so much as bad habits in your daily routine. The causes of this imbalanced condition lie in the diet.

Constipation is caused, in part, by a lack of roughage in the diet — a constant diet of cooked refined foods, all usually seasoned with refined white table salt. On such a diet, sooner or later the intestinal tract becomes irritated and inflamed. Then the valves begin swelling and closing. The entire intestinal tract is blocked by debris of waste matter that failed to pass. Together with mucus, it eventually hardens like cement against the walls of the intestines and, like pipes filled with hardened plaque, waste matter becomes increasingly difficult to pass. The diet must be changed. Raw food and fiber must be added to act as a broom sweeping the system clean.

Although most of us will continue to eat some portion of cooked food in our diet, refined and processed foods should be a thing of the past. The human body was never meant to absorb this deplorable dead substance. It becomes a slow poison. Seldom does the body die suddenly. It slowly succumbs to the inpouring of dead food, which settles into every organ, tissue, atom, cell, muscle and joint until finally the body, magnificent instrument of the spirit that it is, gives up the battle against toxic poison.

Vast hordes of youngsters begin their lives on baby foods in cans or jars, saturated with white sugar, dyes and chemicals. Even before maturity, death has struck in the colon and intestines. Constipation becomes a habit. Parasites and bacteria become rooted in the intestines and colon and the body begins its slow march toward degeneration. The only way purification can occur is through a switch to natural foods, preferably raw for a while. Out of your cupboard must go the refined white sugar, refined white flour, refined white salt, and all the canned and processed foods. In their place must come whole grain flour, natural raw honey, date sugar, and vegetable or mineral salt. The processed foods must be replaced by fresh vegetables and fruits. The diet must include large raw salads, both vegetables and fruits.

You have been brainwashed to believe you must daily fill your body with high quantities of protein, which in itself causes disaster. Too much protein creates a breakdown of the tissues, mucus throughout the bowels, bacteria and parasites breeding throughout the intestinal system. After discarding the processed foods and switching to raw salads, steamed fresh vegetables, fresh fruit, whole grains, plant protein, and protein from dairy products, our first line of defense is to correct constipation*.

Professor Arnold Ehret, in his book *Mucusless Diet Healing System* said: "Every disease, no matter what name it is known by medical science, is constipation, a clogging up of the entire pipe system of the human body. Any special symptom is therefore merely an extraordinary local constipation by more accumulated mucus at this particular place." Aging of the body is the direct result of waste products stored in the cells, tissues, muscles and nerves. Thus if we desire to remain youthful and vital, we must be aware of eliminating the poisonous wastes.

Wastes are eliminated through four distinct channels:

1) the intestinal or digestive tract which involves liver and gallbladder;
2) lungs or respiratory tract;
3) skin;
4) kidneys or urinary tract.

Considering the first, elimination through the intestinal tract, there is a popular belief that it is quite all right to eliminate waste products once a day, but this is not true. Elimination *should* occur as often as food is consumed, three times a day. With only one elimination during twenty-four hours, wastes are retained too long in the intestinal tract, resulting in reabsorption of poisons. These poisons, seeping into every cell, tissue and muscle of the body, float throughout the bloodstream.

The usual procedure is the use of laxatives, which can be extremely dangerous, for most laxatives are in themselves poisonous. It requires considerable effort for the body to eliminate the poison in the laxative. Though it seems to be "moving" your bowels, much of the poison

*See *The Book of Beginning Again*.

enters the bloodstream. Most laxatives contain the metal *mercury* — which is a virulent poison — and artificial citric acids, dyes and sucrose. Many contain phenolphthalein, which is an irritant to the intestinal tract and quite harmful. Taking laxatives to remove accumulated poisons is using poison to remove poison. Continued use will weaken intestinal walls, destroy countless billions of life cells, and upset any natural peristaltic rhythm. Cells destroyed by laxatives enter the bloodstream as more poison creating a vicious cycle — the body attempting valiantly to overcome the effects of laxative poisons. Only general depletion and lowered power of resistance can result.

Constipation can be overcome in only one way. Change to the proper foods, change your source of drinking water, your mental attitude, and begin correct exercising. It requires no magic and no miracles. Here are helpful suggestions:

1) Add fiber foods to your diet. Fruits, vegetables, steel cut oatmeal, bran, grain breads, etc. An excellent choice is jumbo, pitted, unsulfured prunes, purchased at your health store and soaked overnight. Or prune juice. Or stewed prunes before going to bed. Or flaxseed, ground or whole, which is a natural food laxative. Or try eating celery with each meal.

2) In the beginning of your purification program, if you are accustomed to laxatives, you may need to resort to small enemas for a short time. Although they are harmful, they are much to be preferred over laxatives. Fermenting food material must not remain in the colon. Therefore, enemas or internal baths are advisable, but they must not be allowed to become habitual. More about this later.

3) It is well to add some form of soured milk to your diet, such as yogurt, kefir or buttermilk. They help prevent intestinal putrefaction. Or take acidophilus tablets. Hanna Kroeger makes available an excellent product called *Taurin-dophilus*.

4) Eliminate sweet milk at mealtime. It counteracts the action of hydrochloric acid in the digestive juices. Mixing sweet milk with protein also prevents calcium from being distributed into the bloodstream. It then passes out as waste. When the body loses the necessary calcium intake it becomes deficient in one of its most important healing properties. Many who drink sweet milk with protein meals think they are obtaining their required intake of calcium when, actually, the opposite is occurring. Therefore, choose some form of soured milk at meal time. If all forms of milk give you indigestion problems, try raw goat's milk. Its constitution seems more easily digested.

5) Take odorless garlic oil or tablets, an excellent remedy for flatulence. Its natural antibiotic properties neutralize toxins and kill infections.

6) Try bee pollen, which can be purchased at your health store. Its antiputrefactive action is excellent for eliminating gas and killing undesirable bacteria.

7) Add papaya to your meals. Papaya has long been recognized as an aid to protein digestion (meat tenderizers purchased at your supermarket contain considerable papaya). The enzyme, papain, is what makes papaya so effective. It breaks the protein into amino acid, making it more easily assimilated. Why not add a slice of papaya to your lunch and dinner plate? It is excellent to aid digestion and mixes well with fruits, vegetables, nuts, and grains. If you are a meat eater it is even more advisable.

8) And why not add chili powder to some of your food. It is excellent for stimulating the digestive processes. Its best source is cayenne pepper. If it proves too "fiery," purchase it as cayenne herbal capsules from your health store and take it during or immediately after a meal. Cayenne not only stimulates the digestive processes but has many other beneficial side effects. Since it also stimulates blood circulation, it aids arthritis victims. It is a natural diuretic, stimulating the kidneys. Like garlic, it is a powerful enemy of toxicity.

9) Another aid to digestion is the herb peppermint — it also alkalizes an overacid system. A cup of peppermint tea offers instant relief from stomach distress. On a continuing basis try chamomile tea.

10) For the distress of gas try charcoal capsules, available at your health store.

11) Fresh pineapple is a natural aid to digestion, as well as papaya. It contains natural digestive enzymes that aid in digesting meats, cheese and other proteins. It also contains organic iodine to stimulate a sluggish thyroid.

12) If you believe all those television commercials, you are thoroughly convinced that gas and indigestion problems are caused by excessive stomach acid. Apparently many are brainwashed to believe just that, since millions reach for millions of antacid tablets daily hoping to combat stomach distress. But in many cases just the opposite is the problem — too little acid, not too much. The natural condition of the stomach is acid. Hydrochloric acid is poured continuously into the stomach of a healthy body.

When indigestion problems develop it may mean there is an insufficient level of hydrochloric acid. Many suffer from this deficiency, especially older people who have been eating the wrong diet for many years. Instead of reaching for an antacid tablet next time you have stomach distress, try reaching for a hydrochloric acid tablet just prior to or after a meal. Or try sipping, with your meals, a cup of water containing one or two teaspoons of apple cider vinegar and one or two teaspoons of honey. Or water with lemon. You may find your digestion improving considerably.

Also change your eating habits. *Stop eating so fast and do not overeat.* Begin a program of exercise which will enable your body better to produce its own supply of hydrochloric acid. After you take the hydrochloric acid tablet, if you experience a burning sensation in your stomach area, it indicates you do not need the hydrochloric acid tablet and you must search elsewhere for the cause of your digestive problem, the flatulence, the constipation. Try digestive enzyme tablets from your health store. Or cut the acid tablet in half and try again.

13) Don't exercise after eating. Digestive juices are active. Physical activity could cause the gastric juices to back up into the esophagus. Pain! Rest after meals is best, if possible.

14) Heartburn, once triggered, can begin a cycle of asthma attacks. The "bronchodilator" spray which opens bronchial passages during an asthma attack can cause heartburn, which may have triggered the attack in the first place. It's a heartburn-asthma cycle. Again, try resting after meals to give your digestive juices a chance to digest your food. Even try some relaxing tapes, perhaps subliminal, to aid digestion and relaxation. And do be aware that you may need digestive enzymes. Try the papaya, pineapple and raw chlorophyll food enzymes rather than hydrochloric acid. If heartburn continues, try the hydrochloric acid test to see if digestion improves.

15) Jewelry turning black on your fingers and neck? You are overacid. Nitrizine or litmus paper tests of urine showing too yellow? You are overacid. But don't rush for alkalizers from your drugstore which have harmful side effects. Reach instead for a plate of steamed asparagus. Be sure it is a part of your diet for a few days. It is not only an excellent method of alkalizing your system, but is far more pleasant than the usual drugs. The urine will smell like ammonia. That's because the asparagus is causing the system to discharge an oversupply of acidity. Also, garlic tablets or a fresh clove of garlic taken at bedtime acts as an aid to neutralizing the system. A further aid is to take a warm bath and add a cup of baking soda. Do not overdo this aid, however. Too much baking soda bathing can rob the body of too much acid.

Developing Regularity

Form the habit of evacuating at the same time every day to encourage bowel motion. Sit on the stool at the same time whether you have the inclination or not. Do not strain. Simply sit a few moments, gently encouraging the bowels to perform. Manipulate and massage the entire abdomen from right to left. This is the natural movement of waste matter. It passes through the colon from right to left and exits to the rectum from the left side. Manipulating and massaging the abdomen daily is most helpful. Begin the self-massage over the bowels and stomach, kneading them in a circular fashion. Begin low down on the right side, travel up the ascending colon, across the transverse colon and down the other side. Continue this circular massage for a few minutes with both hands. Apply a kneading action. This encourages peristaltic muscular movement and elimination. The body will begin to respond until a good habit is formed. It is well to have the toilet seat as low as possible. If it is too high, place a box under the feet. Better still, find a wide-mouthed container — such as an old wok — to use temporarily as your toilet. Rather than colonics, some may prefer a method of flushing the alimentary canal. This treatment consists of drinking moderately hot water first thing in the morning in combination with special exercises. Hot water drinking is not a new idea. The trouble with those who try it is that they usually do not drink enough. The ideal plan calls for drinking from one to two quarts or more, one or two cups at a time, at intervals of perhaps five minutes, with exercises performed during the intervals.

The water should not be too hot, just enough for one to be able to drink it down rapidly. No one can consume two quarts or more of water in this way in the course of 30 or 40 minutes without accomplishing a very thorough and effective flushing of the alimentary canal. As a means of relief from constipation it is far superior to the usual colon flushing system — the colonic. It is a more natural method. This is not a constipation cure. It is a constipation preventive, and that means a great deal more. A cure means a remedial measure for a condition in which harm has already been accomplished. A preventive is the measure which keeps one in such perfect condition that no disturbance of bodily functions and no poisoning or injury to the body can be accomplished. This particular plan gives one an appetite such as cannot be obtained from any tonic or stomach stimulant.

Incidentally, the general effects are most remarkable in improving the complexion, making the skin smooth, clearing the voice, and in so improving the powers of assimilation that those who are emaciated can regain normal weight, plus perfect digestion. Some prefer to add fresh lemon juice to the water, if the urine tests acid (yellow) with the nitrizine paper test. If it tests alkaline (purple), add a bit of apple cider vinegar. If you can't manage so much water, just drink one large glass of warm lemon water before breakfast.

"An apple a day keeps the doctor away" is a tried and true adage. An apple a day also keeps constipation away and keeping constipation away can certainly keep the doctor away. The organic pectin in the apple does the trick as pectin produces a double action in the intestinal area. If one is suffering from diarrhea the pectin in an apple can bring it under control. On the other hand, an apple can produce the opposite effect, a better bowel movement. Whether or not you have elimination problems, make apples an important part of your diet. Should you eat the skins? Certainly — but only after the apples are washed in Clorox water or vinegar water, or Shaklee's Basic H, or Amway's LOC, to remove chemical spray, paraffin wax and all pollutants. The skin possesses fiber needed for beneficial action in the intestines. It is well to eat apples at bedtime. Hypoglycemics should mix the fruit with a bit of protein — a small chunk of raw natural cheese or a bit of health store organic peanut butter. Eating wheat germ with fruit is also an excellent corrective.

Suggestions to Consider

Never drink coffee or herb teas too hot. And never drink iced beverages. They shock the entire system, especially the digestive system. They should never ever be consumed at mealtime. They stop the entire digestive process and can create considerable digestive problems. The fats in the food are solidified by the iced liquid before the digestive process can break them down, and the solidified fat particles pass into the liver as cholesterol. The liver, reacting, releases great quantities of its own natural cholesterol to meet the invading enemy of fat — so that the entire bloodstream is saturated with disastrous cholesterol. Iced water paralyzes the digestive process. The same is true of hot coffee, which frequently follows a meal. It numbs the nerve control, and the food which may have tasted so delicious will only be partially digested. The rest will lie like waste debris, first in the stomach and then in the rest of the system as it passes through the process of elimination. The stomach was not built to accommodate iced or overly hot liquids, especially with meals when the digestive juices should be most active.

Giving a child, overheated with playing and exercising, a glass of cold liquid is a shock to the entire nervous system, including the stomach. It cannot be properly assimilated and very much disturbs the digestive process for later food intake. The temperature change with anything too hot or too cold is a shock that is difficult to overcome. Repeated daily, the perpetual shock sets up a permanent paralysis of the stomach glands so that later one fails to produce the important hydrochloric acid, pepsin, and digestive juices. Then the entire digestive process needs outside help, such as hydrochloric acid tablets, etc.

If you have already damaged your stomach so that you have ulcers, diverticulitis, or stomach spasms, you may find relief by taking two tablespoons of aloe vera in a little water several times a day. It is very healing and will also stimulate the paralyzed digestive glands. Other herbs which benefit a problem stomach are comfrey, murdock root, damiana leaves, chamomile, and fennel.

Strict food experts advise against combining fruit and vegetables at the same meal. They require different digestive enzymes, even though some stomachs seem to handle them compatibly. In order to avoid digestive problems, it is best to eat them separately. Combining foods that are incompatible results in mucus in the stomach. Even though the stomach requires some mucus, too much prevents the food magnets from reaching their destination. Thus, one may be well fed but suffering from malnutrition.*

Another reason is that it is very difficult to assimilate the chlorophyll of the vegetables with the acids of the fruit — and the fruits all contain acids. The body very badly needs the chlorophyll in the greens. Thus if you mix your greens with your fruit the body is robbed of its chlorophyll. Chlorophyll is probably the most lacking element in any diet. It is wise not to interfere with the assimilation of this important substance. As your body becomes increasingly purified, your digestion becomes so superb that the body will begin to manufacture protein from chlorophyll by combining with the oxygen you inbreathe. That's a safety valve nature built into the body. That is why raw salads and vegetable juices are so important. They produce a lot of chlorophyll in the body. Papaya is the only fruit compatible with vegetables. It could be added to any meal to aid digestion.

The Bean Therapy — As more and more people turn to less meat in the diet, beans are growing in popularity.

*For further information concerning food combining see *The Book of Beginning Again*.

With many, beans "don't get respect." But the proof of their effectiveness is changing that. Beans, together with corn or cornbread, are perfect protein. Vegetarian or not, make beans an important part of your diet. Be sure to soak them overnight, discarding the soak water and adding fresh for cooking. Add onion, a vegetable bullion cube, Real Salt, perhaps a tad of garlic. Add anything else that appeals to you, such as seasoning with pepper sauce when eating — but be sure to eat corn along with them, either cornbread, corn tortillas, corn chips, or corn on the cob. Otherwise beans are not a complete protein food. They are great in a reducing diet because they are low in calories, filled with fiber, and good carbohydrates. If refined white salt is avoided and a good mineral salt added instead, they are excellent to bring down high blood pressure. A sprinkle of pepper-sauce when serving aids in digesting beans.

Do eat a lot of beans: pink, red, pinto, navy, butter beans. Beans of all kind are excellent to maintain energy and blood sugar. Enjoy a bowl for dinner, along with corn-bread and a large salad — a perfect meal for thinning the blood, reducing cholesterol, improving circulation, controlling blood pressure, warding off diabetes and controlling blood sugar levels. Add garlic to the beans near the end of or after cooking. Garlic's high sulfur content will help prevent heart attack, blood clots, hardening of arteries, strokes, arthritis, inflammation, hypoglycemia, anemia and infections.

Cereal Grains — must be unprocessed. Avoid the usual cold processed breakfast cereals like the plague. The label on the box may describe the contents as wheat, corn, rice or oats, but the cereal dumped into the breakfast bowl is often far removed from the original product. Most contain little more nourishment than boiled wallpaper, since they have been so processed — not only that, but they contain many chemicals with the sparkling white sugar added for "energy," making them "new and improved." A few exceptions may be found at your health store. Also there are now appearing cereals without sugar. Try Oat Bran, Grape Nuts, Shredded Wheat, with date sugar and Mocha Milk. Read labels. The cereal industry is becoming aware of the health trend in America and may begin producing healthy items. Steel cut oatmeal cooked with raisins and eaten with date sugar and Mocha Milk is excellent. Steel cut oatmeal is usually available only at health stores.

Helping a Distressed Infant — To help an infant constantly vomiting after each feeding, try this old German recipe: Dissolve a spoonful of potato starch or cornstarch in cold water. Bring to boil a cup of half-milk half-water (raw unhomogenized milk). While stirring the boiling mixture, drop in as much potato starch or cornstarch as needed to create a semi-thick fluid. After allowing it to cool to lukewarm, give 1/2 to one teaspoon to the infant five minutes before each feeding. The semi-thick starch fluid relaxes the nerves of the stomach, allowing the infant to digest the feeding. After about two weeks the problem should be ended, but if not, continue the procedure until relief is noticed. But do not continue longer then necessary. Cornstarch is not advisable over a long period. If it doesn't help the problem, try agar-agar from the health store.

The Enema or Internal Bath — If you have been constipated for a long time and using laxatives intermittently, the walls of your intestines probably are coated with a hard crust of matter resembling limestone in an old water pipe, so that the opening through which the fecal matter must pass is greatly reduced. The same is true in the case of arteriosclerosis or hardening of the arteries. The arteries through which your blood passes becomes hardened.

The intestines, like the arteries, contain countless little ducts which spread along the walls of the stomach and intestines. If the walls of the intestines are coated with hardened waste matter it is impossible for nutritive substances of food to enter the lymphatic and bloodstreams which carry them to all parts of the system. Even should you choose to eat the proper kind of food, your system cannot assimilate its good "fuel." The body may be undergoing a slow process of starvation and self-poisoning. It may be wise to seek a colonic expert for a few oxygen-colonic treatments, but it is not wise to continue them for an extended period. You may prefer your own enema.

How often an enema may be needed depends entirely upon your condition. Frequently a daily enema is advisable for a week or ten days, then three times a week, then twice, then once until it is no longer needed. During this time your change of diet will be helping your body to discard its impurities. It will also be aiding in loosening the hardened fecal matter along intestinal walls. Use the enema as long as necessary, but not one day longer. Do not form the habit. It is used simply to help nature at the beginning of your purification program. Add a teaspoon of salt. Or the juice of a lemon, which cuts away accumulated phlegm. Or add diluted grape juice which feeds natural acidophilus bacilli into the lower bowels. Occasionally add coffee. A coffee enema performs wonders.

Constipation must ultimately be overcome by correct diet. As you taper off the enemas, try using only a pint to loosen congested matter at the base of the rectum. This action will not be habit forming and will allow the natural peristaltic movement to occur without the aid of additional water.

The Flaxseed Therapy — Before breakfast, take at least one heaping teaspoon of flaxseed, either whole or finely ground. Drink it with room-temperature distilled water, followed by at least one large glass of warm water. Flaxseed may be finely ground in a small electric Moulinex nut grinder (found at your health store). Grind only enough for a week's supply, after which any ground seeds should be discarded since the oil of the seeds becomes rancid. Flaxseed is not a direct laxative. Like prunes, it is a food containing natural laxative properties, thus making it a natural means of helping the body discard wastes. It is quite safe to take flaxseed habitually, since it is a natural food. In the intestinal tract it forms a gelatinous bulk, which acts upon the peristaltic activity of the intestines, helping to bring about natural evacuation. The "jelly" that is formed coats the lining of the stomach, healing irritations, inflammations and even ulcers. It also breaks up waste debris and cleans the bowels.

You may need to repeat the flaxseed at noon and again just before retiring if you have a stubborn case of constipation. Take a heaping teaspoon with water three times a day until evacuation begins to occur easily. Then cut back gradually to once a day, preferably when rising, and continue for the rest of your life if you wish. It will do no harm and a great deal of good. Always carry ground flaxseed when you travel. More about flaxseed oil later.

You may wish to consider herbs. For inflamed or irritated bowels and intestines, comfrey root, goldenseal, dandelion and chickweed have been found helpful. For diarrhea try slippery elm, thyme, barberry bark. For aids to digestion try fenugreek, ginger, lobelia, peppermint. For gas pains try valerian root, ginger, thyme, sassafras or catnip. For indigestion try ginger root, capsicum, goldenseal, catnip. To destroy tapeworms and roundworms try watermelon seed tea or capsules. Figs are also quite effective in destroying worms in the intestines.

The following exercise will help to begin a natural peristaltic movement to heal or avoid constipation: Lie on your back and bring the knees up, clasping your arms around them. Pump the abdominal muscles in and out, pressing against the legs.

An Aid To Reducing — For a reducing diet I can heartily recommend a teaspoon or tablespoon of flaxseed, either whole or ground, taken with a large glass of water half an hour before meals. The gelatinous mass which expands in the stomach is more than adequate to discourage the intake of large meals. And it's a perfect food in itself. No dangerous chemicals added. It not only is an excellent means of reducing, but performs all sorts of other good actions — it breaks up encrusted wastes along intestinal walls, it establishes regular bowel movements, it absorbs toxins in the bloodstream and flushes them out. The natural oil in the flaxseed absorbs the "bad" oil in the diet and carries it out of the system — and it breaks up oil and cholesterol deposits in the arteries which lead to heart attacks. If heavy dosage proves too much for your system, either cut down the intake or take it only once a day before your largest meal.

Another plant fiber excellent for slimming is *guar gum* available at your health store. If a teaspoonful of guar gum is taken daily with a glass of water half an hour before a meal, it expands in the stomach and creates a clear fiber gel that makes one feel full. The fiber is not absorbed into the bloodstream but is eliminated through the digestive processes. Its gel also prevents the absorption of fats through the intestines. Ask for *Bioguar* or *Theraguar* at your health store.

Healing a Wounded Colon

When the colon becomes ill this is the beginning of severe health problems. The best approach to health is first to change the diet, as has already been outlined. For a while you may need to be on a raw food diet of fruits, vegetables, seeds, nuts, yeast flakes, raw milk in moderation, raw cheese in moderation, sprouts. It was once felt colitis required a "soft food" diet — poached eggs, creamed soups, steel cut oatmeal, cottage cheese, stewed fruits. You may be convinced this approach is best. If so, proceed. But avoid the Jellos, the processed foods, the white flour, sugar, salt products. And *do* eat raw salads, beginning with small portions if necessary. They are the finest of all natural healers. And do eat citrus fruits to help break up encrusted phlegm.

Eat a small amount of yogurt or take some kind of acidophilus culture to restore natural flora or friendly bacteria to intestines. So long as intestinal walls are clogged with cement-like waste debris — cholesterol or impacted oils and fats — regardless how pure your diet may be, the nutritional quality cannot be absorbed into your system. It is because of this we frequently recommend tinctures of vitamins and minerals, dropped under the tongue. They will be absorbed by the system that is weakened with toxic wastes when vitamins, minerals and enzymes from its food intake cannot be absorbed. I can recommend Fanie's Sublingual products (address elsewhere) as a splendid source. Then make sure of elimination by using any of the following suggestions:

1) Consider the flaxseed I've already mentioned.

2) Take one or two tablespoons of psyllium powder a day in four ounces of water or juice. It can be purchased at a health store. It may be taken at bedtime or when rising, at either time followed by a full glass of distilled water. It forms a soft bulk in the intestinal tract. As it moves through the digestive system it becomes a gelatin-like substance, gathering into itself much of the hardened fecal debris in pockets all along intestines and colon. Its mysterious substance seems to absorb much hardened, impacted waste that may have lain in pockets in intestines and colon for years. As this debris is softened and coaxed out of the pockets, psyllium will then proceed to heal the wounds. If psyllium powder seems too severe, switch to the flaxseed program. Jason Winters offers a product called *Colon Cleanser*, available at health stores. It's absolutely marvelous. Whether constipated or not, you should take this or a similar colon cleanser at regular intervals to make sure waste toxins do not accumulate in the colon.

3) Following the days of taking the psyllium, it may be well to take slippery elm herbs in capsules.

4) Eat a lot of okra if it is in season.

5) Since goldenseal herb capsules and garlic are both natural antibiotics it is well to also take them to prevent any infection developing.

6) A daily tablet of vitamin B6 might be advisable.

7) You may wish to take 4 to 6 ounce doses of liquid pectin three times a day to discover if it aids your digestive function.

8) *Whey* possesses a unique ability to cleanse the

urinary tract, simultaneously stimulating a cleansing flow of urine.

9) Try clay capsules, which are reputed to purify the entire intestinal tract, often available at your health store. If not, order from Tammlyn Products. (address elsewhere)

Kundalini and Elimination — Since we always consider "the whole being" we must consider the spiritual aspects, even in such a mundane function as waste elimination. At the base of the spine is the sacred life brain, or kundalini, from which flows the creative life energies. When the colon is filled with waste matter, there is pressure upon this great sacral plexus, closing off the flow of life-giving energy throughout the body — which is an excellent reason the colon should be emptied at least twice daily. When waste products congest in the colon, gas is formed throughout the intestinal tract, and seeps into muscles, cells, lungs, heart and brain. Waste product poisons are thus settled in these tissues and organs. When the flow of life energy is cut off from the body's other energy centers, not only does disease result, but mental functions are depressed and spiritual unfoldment is curtailed.

Chapter Five

The Liver, Alcoholism, Hypoglycemia

The liver is the largest gland in your body. It's called a gland because it secretes and excretes substances. Like the heart, the liver is never at rest. It is perpetually receiving or releasing various foods, chemicals, hormones, bile, fats, vitamins, poisons. It's a chemical factory, a purifying powerhouse, a storage house, a laboratory — all of extreme importance.

It is involved with digestion, fully cooperating with the gall bladder and pancreas. It possesses the unique quality of regeneration, meaning that if it is seriously damaged through infectious viruses, diet, alcohol, poison, drug abuse, if given the opportunity through a purification program, it will or can possibly heal itself of the damage and restore itself to wholeness. It cannot, of course, if the abuse is continued over too long a period. But once liver damage becomes obvious, if the patient is willing to seek a purifying approach, the liver, seeming to possess a psychic sense, will struggle toward complete regeneration.

The liver is the body's busiest organ. It's the liver that forms the bile necessary for proper digestion. The function of bile is to emulsify fats and thus permit their normal absorption from the small intestine. A human produces about two quarts of this vital substance each day. Actually, the liver absorbs over-aged blood cells and, from their hemoglobin, produces the yellowish bile fluid which is then stored in the gall bladder. Most of the bile, so necessary for digestion, is used over and over again. From the gall bladder it is sent into the intestine where it is absorbed by the blood and then dispatched again to the liver. A damaged or infected liver fails to produce or recycle the bile. When this happens, hepatitis or yellow jaundice may occur, the skin turning yellow because of a malfunctioning in the marvelous liver/gall bladder mechanical machinery.

The liver is a "clearing-house" for all the foods you digest. The liver decides which is the "chaff" and which is the "wheat." It retains the proper amounts of nutritional elements from your food. The rest is deposited into the intestine and bloodstream as waste — much as a juicer separates the juice from the pulp.

Avoid routine immunization injections which are supposed to guard you against both of the main types of hepatitis. They may have within themselves hidden carriers of disease. Instead, develop the habit of washing your hands thoroughly after the bathroom. Keep the bathroom scrupulously clean. However, if your doctor suspects hepatitis, a vaccine to prevent transfer of the infection is available. He will first take a blood test to determine if you are already infected. The blood test will also reveal whether you already have enough antibodies to be immune to the virus. Usually hepatitis B heals itself and the virus is slowly eliminated from the body. In some rare cases the virus lingers as a "hidden" infection. Women planning motherhood would do well to ask for a blood test to reveal whether or not a hepatitis infection is present, because a hidden infection is often transferred to infants during delivery.

There are several methods of damaging the liver:

1) virus infection, sometimes resulting in hepatitis;
2) cirrhosis of the liver, caused principally by alcoholism and wrong diet;
3) obesity;
4) drug abuse.

Hepatitis — Infectious hepatitis is an acute infection of the liver and is often traced to fecal contamination of water, to polluted water systems and through contaminated foods. If this virus enters the digestive tract of a susceptible person the disease breaks out in ten to forty days. The virus can live for months in a tiny speck on a toilet seat, be picked up on the hand and enter the mouth on any food held in the same hand.

Serum hepatitis, on the other hand, has been detected only in blood and is usually transmitted through blood transfusions (which is why I have warned against blood transfusion in previous writings). It may also be transmitted through unsterilized medical instruments or unsanitary inoculation methods. The first symptoms hit suddenly — violent headaches, nausea, tiredness, chills, vomiting, cramps in the upper right part of the abdomen, loss of appetite and an itchy skin. The next symptom is the onslaught of jaundice. Jaundice is an acute disease indicating that the liver is filtering excessive poisons, pollutions and toxins. The skin turns yellow or even orange or green. Even though you may look ghastly after jaundice occurs, you will begin to feel better, since the skin discoloration indicates the capillaries of the liver are no longer blocked.

The infected bile, produced by the liver which previously had backed up into the blood, is now released into the bloodstream and is passing out of the body. The discoloration may continue for a few days or several months. Bed rest is strongly advised. Recovery is gradual. Since most of the drugs now used against hepatitis have incredible side effects, it may seem better to let nature take its course. Change to a vegetarian raw food diet, do not overeat and get plenty of bed rest. Take sensible doses of vitamin C along with a program of vitamin-mineral tablets, especially the B vitamins. Drink several glasses of lemon water daily — a full glass of distilled water with the juice of a fresh lemon. Add honey if desired, in moderation. Cease this activity if the system becomes over-alkaline. Use nitrizine paper, available from drug or health store, to test the urine.

Treatments of hepatitis and other liver disorders begin with *dandelion root* herb capsules or eaten as a green vegetable. Dandelion stimulates bile production, combats toxins, reduces a swollen liver, corrects jaundice and treats chronic hepatitis. *Cascara sagrada* is renowned for treating liver disorders and gall stones. It's an excellent natural laxative. *Licorice root*, second only to ginseng in Chinese herbalism, is recognized as the great detoxifier. Its diuretic properties aid in treating liver disorders. It reduces the accumulation of triglycerides in the liver, increases glycogen levels, prevents cirrhosis, and treats hepatitis B.

Whereas hepatitis was once rare, it seems to be fairly common now. So much so that one may wish to use preventive measures. Dr. Kurt Donsbock, famous among holistic adherents, offers a licorice liver tonic called *glycyrrhisin*. We have long known licorice to have an anti-inflammatory and detoxicating effect not only upon the liver but the entire body. We women recognize it too as an aid to female problems. If you've had a flare-up of the liver, including even chronic viral hepatitis, do contact Dr. Donsbock and inquire about his licorice liver tonic. Telephone (619)428-8585. But don't stay on licorice too long, it can increase heart problems.

Cirrhosis — A prolonged diet of damaging food results in cirrhosis, which is actually a process of liver cells dying off faster than the organ can regenerate itself. The dead cells, rather than being replaced by vigorous live cells, are replaced by more dead cells containing a hard, fibrous center of connective tissue. As these cells increase they form a mass of hardened dead structure incapable of carrying out all the vast laboratory activities once handled by an active liver. The result is death of the body through the body's own poisons.

Alcoholism and Low Blood Sugar — Dr. Som, the naturopath who taught me so much about natural healing methods, and who was quoted so much in *The Book of Beginning Again*, considered alcoholism a disease. Let's talk first about the effect of alcohol in the body. Alcohol is a carbohydrate made up of carbon, hydrogen and oxygen, differing in arrangement from molecules in other carbohydrates. It acts as a fuel for heat and power but provides nothing to the maintenance of the body. Alcohol is a depressant. One gets the impression of being stimulated because of a temporary rise in blood sugar, but the stimulation is false because it only temporarily dilates the miniature blood vessels on the surface of the skin, creating a sensation of warmth. Alcohol kills appetite, causing the alcoholic to become undernouished.

Alcoholics are the victims of low blood sugar which

means too much insulin, the direct opposite of diabetes which has too little insulin. Too much insulin is created by the adrenals and the pituitary. The pituitary fails to stimulate the adrenal-cortical gland, creating a deficiency in adrenal-cortical hormones. The answer to the problem could lie in the diet — making sure the diet regulates the blood sugar so that it does not fall below safe levels. The diet should be high in fat and plant protein and low in undesirable carbohydrates. Often, the alcoholic reaches for a drink subconsciously to raise the blood sugar. Low blood sugar in turn causes the alcoholic to crave alcohol.

It is generally felt that a diet rich in vitamins and minerals will balance the blood sugar, and the functioning of adrenal glands and pituitary. It may require massive doses of vitamins A, C, D and E and all of the B vitamins until the alcoholic experiences no need for the effect of alcohol. The carbohydrates to be avoided are the white sugars, white flours, refined white salt, processed foods, pies, cakes, ice cream, caffeine, sweet custards, puddings, tea (not herbal teas), potatoes, rice, grapes, raisins, plums, figs, dates, bananas, spaghetti, macaroni, noodles, wines, cordials, cocktails and beer. It is presumed that some of these items may be returned to the diet slowly as the patient recovers from his need for alcohol — such as potatoes, rice, bananas, and noodles.

The good carbohydrates are vegetables and fruits. Avoid, too, animal fats and focus on "good" fats, such as flaxseed oil or cod liver oil. And use virgin olive oil or canola in cooking and in salads.

When a child is given a diet containing white flour (even D-vitaminized) and sugar and homogenized milk, his vitamin deficiency grows steadily worse, creating adrenal disorders and a malfunctioning of the pituitary. As he nears maturity his blood sugar level is held alarmingly low, creating a desire and craving for fulfillment, usually in the form of alcohol which creates an instantaneous rise in blood sugar. The alcoholic is literally starving for food which his diet is not supplying. Often a glandular balance is disturbed because of constant anxiety, a nervous disorder, or stress. Here again, the victim often turns to alcohol to fill the requirements his body needs and in which his diet is deficient.

What we are saying is that if an alcoholic is fed with a proper diet and given the proper vitamins and minerals, there is every possibility that he will completely recover from alcoholism and live a happy, normal life.

To regulate a low blood sugar problem (hypoglycemia) it may be temporarily necessary for you to eat a bite of food every two hours. Check your attitude. Do you harbor a repressed hate and apparently insolvable frustration, an intolerable personal dilemma? Do you suddenly break out in tears for no reason whatsoever? Watch your diet concerning blood sugar. Counseling and many books are available to help with this problem.

Obesity — In the majority of obese patients, tests invariably indicate some measure of liver abnormality. The diet — sweets, processed carbohydrates, overconsumption of flesh food, "junk foods" — is much involved in the ongoing operation of the liver. It *can* be damaged beyond its ability to regenerate itself.

Drug Abuse — Drugs given a patient by a doctor are often a paramount source of liver damage, especially the antibiotics. Aureomycin is especially noted as extremely hazardous. Also sulfa drugs. When accepting a prescription for a drug from a doctor, be sure to ask him to read the list of possible side effects as they are listed in his medical dictionary. It is obvious, of course, that hallucinogenic drugs may be damaging.

The Liver Fast and Gallstones — Dr. Som often prescribed the following for restoring the liver and passing gallstones:

The first day, on arising, drink a glass of warm water with fresh lemon juice added (1/2 lemon). Two hours later, for breakfast, eat all you want of stewed tomatoes and drink tomato juice. Alternate between the warm water-lemon juice, and the stewed tomatoes and tomato juice every two hours for one day, two days, or three until you feel your system is purified. To stew the tomatoes, peel, cut up and add a little distilled water, a little seasoning salt and onions. They should be simmered slowly. Do not add fat or oil of any kind. At bedtime of the last day prepare the following: 3 oz. pure olive oil, 3 oz. cold pressed castor oil and 3 oz. whipped cream. These cold pressed oils are available from Dr. McGarey's A.R.E. Clinic in Phoenix, Cayce Corner. (See last chapter for address.) Or from your health food store. Some supermarkets now carry cold pressed olive oil.

Drink it just before retiring and lie quite still for at least half an hour so you do not become nauseated. You may place a large book on the abdomen to hold the stomach steady. It is important to keep this mixed oil-cream cocktail down. Sometime during the night you will eliminate considerable poisons or the gallstones in the stool. After this, you may break the fast, but in any event do not continue it beyond three days. If you simply cannot ingest the total of six ounces of the castor or olive oil, then take at least three ounces of either oil or mixed oils. It's the oil which will eliminate the stones easily, softening them enough so that passage will not be painful.

Jason Winters, in his book *Killing Cancer*, offers a similar treatment. Drink one quart of apple juice daily for five days to soften gallstones. On the sixth day, skip dinner and at six p.m. take a tablespoon of Epsom salts with water. Repeat at eight p.m. At ten p.m. make a cocktail of four ounces olive oil and four ounces of fresh squeezed lemon juice. (Dr. Som suggested grapefruit juice when he taught of this same remedy). Shake vigorously and drink. Go to bed immediately. Again place a heavy item such as a telephone book or large dictionary on the stomach and lie very still for at least an hour. In the morning the softened gallstones should pass.

Silymarin — a common seed, is being hailed as a superb liver fortifier. It's an extract of the milk thistle weed. It's sold in health stores as *Hepatone* or *Lyverene*. Bleeding of the esophagus is sometimes caused by high blood pressure in patients suffering liver disease. *Ethamolin* will often prevent such bleeding. See your doctor.

Chapter Six

You Are What You — Digest

There's an old adage which states that "you are what you eat." But it isn't so. The adage should say "you are what you digest."

Much more is involved in digestion than was once thought. The steps are not simple. They include eating the right food, chewing it properly, absorbing the nutrients, secreting enzymes for proper assimilation, the condition of the digestive tract lining, the perpetual process of elimination. We have already covered some of these activities.

The entire process of digestion begins in the mouth. The food absolutely *must* be chewed thoroughly before it departs for the stomach. This action breaks down the particles and surrounds the food with saliva which contains the enzyme ptyalin. Particularly must starch foods, the grains, be properly salivated. The stomach contains no starch-digesting enzymes. So, much depends on the oral breakdown of starch particles. The small intestines complete the breakdown of starch digestion with pancreatic enzymes, but if they are insufficient, and if the starch food has not been properly salivated in the mouth, problems of digestion develop.

Departing the stomach, the food passes through a valve into the small intestine. Flowing into the intestine along with the food there is, or should be, a supply of pancreatic enzymes to aid digestion. From the liver and gallbladder there should also be a flow of bile. As the food moves along the intestinal canal its molecules should be absorbed through the villi — tiny finger-like projections that line intestinal walls. The food's nutrients pass through the villi into the bloodstream.

The pancreas manufactures three kinds of enzymes and, depending upon the food eaten, secretes the amount necessary for digestion. These three kinds of enzymes digest fat, protein, and carbohydrates. They mix with hydrochloric acid and pepsin in the stomach to digest protein. They unite with bile from the liver/gallbladder to digest fats. The pancreatic enzymes mix with salivary enzymes to digest starches.

The greatest problem of digestion is possibly the fat intake. It is fat which slows the processes. So even though the enjoyment of a meal may be enhanced by added butter, melted cheese or gravy, and sauces made with oil, the digestive processes will suffer. If you enjoy buttered foods, add the butter after the food is on your plate to prevent rancidity through cooking. Even though a recipe calls for cheese while baking, add grated cheese after removing the dish from the oven. This way, the dish will contain the butter or cheese without cooking the fats. Also, instead of butter — let's say on your potato or popcorn — try sesame oil, flaxseed oil, canola, olive oil, or any of the "good" oils from your health store. Add it to your veggies and corn on the cob, too. It really *is* delicious.

The Enzymes: Multiform Chemists

Food could not be assimilated were it not for miracle workers named *enzymes*. All protein is converted into amino acids by the catalytic presence of enzymes. Enzymes are to the body what tools are to the gardener. Enzymes control chemical reaction of food as it is digested and absorbed. They release nutriments as needed for physical and mental activity. They are known by the kind of work they do — some do "spade" work while others carry "trays" of food particles to the chemical laboratories in the liver and pancreas. Vitamins, sometimes called "co-enzymes," are co-partners with enzymes in this work.

Enzymes are furnished principally by raw fruits and vegetables. Cooking usually destroys them. As low a temperature as 99 degrees damages their potency, while 140 degrees destroys all enzymes. Therefore it's important to eat raw foods daily if buoyant health is to be maintained. Again, the old axiom *you are what you eat* is not altogether true. Actually, *you are what you digest*— due to the wonder-working catalytic presence of enzymes.

Enzymes are necessary for biochemical processes to take place in the body. Enzymes themselves cannot remain active without two very important factors — first, organic minerals and second, raw protein. The organic mineral is a co-enzyme called *coferment*. The raw protein factor is called *apoferment*. With these two biocatalysts present the body can make its own enzymes. So there absolutely must be some organic minerals and raw proteins consumed daily for enzymes to be properly formed. Chemicals added to foods destroy raw protein, as does heating and freezing.

Vegetables and fruits not loaded with natural minerals will not supply your need for organic minerals. Kelp tablets taken daily fill the need. Raw proteins include sunflower seeds, bee pollen, raw whole milk, clabbered milk, raw natural cheese, sprouted grains and seeds, raw fresh nuts — almonds, peanuts, Brazil nuts, walnuts — fresh from the shell. Rice polish is rich in raw proteins and organic minerals. Brewer's yeast is an excellent source of raw protein. Whenever possible, purchase organically grown fruits and vegetables that have not been covered with chemical sprays. It is the sprays which prevent organic minerals from producing the important enzymes in your system. Or wash your fruits and vegetables with, say, Amway's LOC, before eating to remove the coating of atmospheric pollutants and sprays.

Too often we are so busily concerned with our vitamin-mineral-protein craze, we overlook the importance of enzymes. But every living cell contains these delicate living substances. Enzymes actually may contain the secret of life itself. It is the enzymes in the seeds which cause them to sprout. It is the enzymes in the human system which makes it possible to digest food, changing it into muscles, nerves, tissues, bones and even new cells. It is the presence of enzymes in saliva which breaks down food constituents even in the mouth and begins the digestive process. They permeate the pancreas, the walls of the stomach and small intestines to create the chemical changes involved in digestion and assimilation of food. They are present in the glands of the endocrine system. In fact, it is the presence of enzymes in every cell of the body that adds to its mysterious life force.

The vitamins and minerals so essential to your well-being could never be assimilated were it not for the presence of enzymes. The enzymes in the cells are continuously and perpetually being depleted. The normal procedure is for the body to manufacture a continuous supply of new enzymes. The full replacement can only occur when the body is functioning at top efficiency.

As the body grows older or becomes increasingly weakened, its ability to produce new and vibrant enzymes is curtailed. As the cells with their enzymes continually die, fewer enzymes are replaced and the replacements are often weaker and less vital. Could the dietary habits of the human race be responsible? Could enzymes be the secret of longevity? Could man improve his well-being by switching to foods containing more live enzymes? In its efforts to carry on the process of digestion and assimilation, the body draws on its reserve supply from nerves, muscles and bloodstream. But just as any reservoir becomes depleted unless its elements are replaced, sooner or later the body's supply of enzymes is diminished, causing an impaired digestive system.

Just as the cells in the human body contain the mysterious enzymes, so do the cells of all plant and animal life. It is the enzymes in plant life that give it its incredible ability to break through soil, and even cement, to find its way toward the life-giving rays of the sun. It is the action of the enzymes that brings about the myriad changes involved in ripening fruit and maturing vegetables. When raw live foods are taken into the system, so also are the invaluable enzymes. The enzymes in raw food, such as salads, quickly replenish the enzymes in human cells.

The cooked food diet of the average American has lost every trace of its original enzyme content. Perhaps this is why drugstores do a thriving business in items which purport to aid digestive problems — those effervescents to relieve the gas caused by the body's inability to digest and assimilate the foods that contain no live enzymes.

One can purchase enzyme tablets at a health store. There are enzymes to digest fat known as *lipase*. Those known as *protease* aid in digesting protein. Those known as *amylase* help digest starches and carbohydrates. They contain trypsin and chymotrypsin. Many who suffer digestive problems find it necessary to take enzyme tablets with each meal — which is certainly wiser than taking the Tums and Di-Gels and the fizzies. Many also find it wise to take hydrochloric acid with their meals — or sip a small glass of water containing two teaspoons of apple cider vinegar, which supplies hydrochloric acid.

There is now available a product called *Co-enzyme 10* which can be purchased at your health store. It may solve many digestive problems. It enhances oxidation; heals damaged tissues; aids in healing ulcers; restores energy; accelerates weight loss; heals periodontal gum tissues; aids in preventing heart disease, high blood pressure, diabetes; and destroys free radicals. Always buy the highest potency possible.

Co-enzyme 10 is used in the treatment of cardiovascular irregularities and disorders. It reduces the risk of heart attack. It has shown significant results in improving conditions of edema, lung congestion and liver swelling. It has been successful in treating gingivitis disorders or gum disease. Its use actually minimizes the ill effects of radiation or chemotherapy treatments. In experiments with laboratory rats it has been found to extend life. Life survival in mice was extended by 56%. In experiments with humans it has been shown to increase energy, prevent toxicity, significantly reduce high blood pressure and aid in preventing aging diseases.

The most natural and effective enzyme known is found in the papaya which contains a protein digestive enzyme called *papain*. It not only aids digestion but detoxifies the system. Why not try a fast from one to three days on nothing but papaya? Have you ever witnessed what papaya tenderizer does to tough meat? Well, it acts similarly inside your digestive tract, which is loaded with hardened protein waste material, usually the result of meat putrefaction over a long period of time. These crystallized toxins may have lain in your intestines for years, slowly hardening in the intracellular spaces. The papaya not only works to dissolve the hardened toxic wastes — the indol, skatol, and phenol which form as islands of putrefaction — but also heals the irritated and inflamed lining of the digestive tract and stomach.

Westerners believe they are fulfilling their protein requirement by overindulging in flesh food. Even a one-day diet on nothing but papaya would do wonders to relieve the overladen digestive system of its burden of putrefied protein. Once the system is cleansed and you are aware that it is wise to eat less than the suggested daily requirement of protein, perhaps your system will begin immediately to respond with better digestion.

Pancreatic enzymes aid in the digestion of all foods but especially protein and starch. Those unable to digest milk would do well to take a pancreatic enzyme tablet. The inability to digest milk indicates the lack of such an enzyme, which is often destroyed by gastric juices in the stomach. Avoid buying the usual pancreatic product since it contains the pancreas of hog meat. Take, instead, *Stilliangia*. It will stimulate the pancreas to produce an increased outflow of its own pancreatic enzymes, an aid to destroying cancer cells. Consider adding a slice of papaya to your dinner plate of cooked food each night or sip a glass of papaya juice.

Medical science and the health seeker are becoming increasingly aware of the importance of enzymes and the result of enzyme deficiencies. When the bloodstream is lacking in minerals or proteins it need not necessarily mean that the diet is deficient in these items. It could mean that the body lacks the ability to properly assimilate food because of enzyme deficiencies.

Often the diet will contain vitamins, minerals and proteins but they fail to reach the bloodstream. Because of a lack of enzymes in the digestive tract the food passes from the body instead of being assimilated through the villi in the intestines into the bloodstream, because the villi are covered by encrusted waste. A diet deficient in raw foods will eventually create such an enzyme deficiency. To repeat, cooked or processed foods contain no enzymes whatsoever since any temperature over 120 degrees Fahrenheit kills them. Vitamins survive quite high temperatures — even canned fruits and vegetables may still contain a rich supply of vitamins. But their enzyme content has been completely destroyed in the canning or cooking process.

Pasteurized milk suffers the same fate. It may still contain its vitamin content but be unassimilable by the human system because the pasteurization process has destroyed the valuable enzymes. Butter and cheese made from pasteurized milk will also be devoid of enzymes. This would point to the value of raw milk, raw sweet butter and raw natural cheese. Cold temperatures also affect the enzyme activity but it does not destroy them. Foods placed in the refrigerator or freezer have their enzymes tentatively inactivated, but restoring the foods to normal temperature restores the enzyme activity.

All this research stipulates that the human race must begin to include a great share of raw food in the diet if it is to survive. The incredible change in the health of zoo animals when switched to raw foods indicates that the human body would similarly respond. There has never been a human ailment — particularly arthritis — that did not respond to a temporary diet of uncooked foods. Complete rehabilitation may necessitate more than a diet, but the dietary change alone has worked wonders. The same is true of every human ailment — improvement and even complete healings are obvious when the switch is made to raw foods.

The experiment with raw foods on cats carried out by Dr. Francis Pottinger in 1946 bears repeating. His report appeared in the August issue of the *American Journal of Orthodontics*. Nine hundred cats were used in his ten-year experiment. Some were given a diet of raw meat, raw milk and cod-liver oil. The cats receiving this raw food diet enjoyed a full life span free of disease, reproducing in a normal manner, the mother cats nursing their young. They displayed an inbuilt resistance to illness, infection and parasites. On the other hand, the cats receiving only cooked meat developed ailments very similar to those of the human family — pneumonia, heart problems, nephritis, paralysis, arthritis, blindness, defective hearing, asthma — all diseases covering the gamut of human misery. They also experienced a high mortality rate. The kittens of the third generation all died within six months. Thus the ten-year experiment came to an enforced end.

During the experiment, Dr. Pottinger substituted pasteurized milk, evaporated milk, sweetened condensed milk for raw milk. Removal of the raw milk created considerable havoc. On the pasteurized and processed milk, bones became soft and many illnesses began to manifest. This experiment could very possibly point to the importance of enzymes in raw food as well as other vital substances as yet undiscovered. Loud will be the cry that the digestive system will seldom tolerate raw foods in quantities because the digestive apparatus has already been considerably damaged. All that can be done in such cases is to try raw fruit and vegetable juices along with cooked foods, until the digestive system improves. More raw vegetables can gradually be added until the full digestive apparatus is restored.

A totally raw food diet is not advisable. It requires thinking almost exclusively about food — and there is more to life than food. All that is urged is that the diet include daily raw salads of either fruit or vegetables along with cooked food. If you eat an all-cooked meal then you should probably take an enzyme tablet *with* the meal to aid digestion, not afterward. If the enzyme is in capsule form, open the capsule and sprinkle the contents on your food. Even raw vegetable salads could be thus supplemented.

Heartburn — is caused when stomach acids back up into the esophagus, a tube through which food passes on its way to the stomach. To avoid the problem, one must avoid foods and actions which relax the sphincter muscular valve which normally prevents the acids from splashing back into the esophagus. Chocolate relaxes the valve so should be avoided. So should all forms of alcohol and fatty foods. Onions and garlic affect some people. Avoid coffee altogether.

Place books or blocks to elevate the head of your bed. This is much preferred over higher pillows. Eat slowly, don't ever overeat, don't snack just before bedtime and don't lie down immediately after eating. Give up cigarettes, especially after a meal. Take Pepto Bismol to protect the burning area. If the pain continues, see a doctor.

Hiatus Hernia — If you *do* suffer from chronic heartburn and the doctor has ruled out ulcers you might have a hiatus hernia. It is a very common ailment and easily treated once you are aware of what is causing your problems. A hiatus hernia is a bulge of the stomach which protrudes into the chest cavity, usually resulting in frequent heartburn. All of the suggestions listed above for heartburn will ease your symptoms. Also try the homeopathic remedy called *Mag Phos*.

Diarrhea — is a condition created when there is such an imbalance in the digestive function, the water content is not properly removed from the food mass in the intestines and both food and water are expelled instead of solid feces. This means little or none of the nutrients from the food is absorbed into the bloodstream, cells, muscles, or glands. A continuation of this situation can lead to a gradual weakening and, carried to its drastic conclusion, even death — death actually through malnutrition or starvation.

Watery stools — *diarrhea* — indicates the presence of malevolent bacteria in the digestive tract and, perhaps, parasites. Or a serious virus infection. Along with the watery stool, all the carbohydrates, fats and many minerals, especially calcium, potassium, iron, phosphorus, are lost. Nor does the body absorb vitamins A, D, K, and E. With the loss of iron, anemia develops. The loss of vitamin A could result in respiratory problems. Hypoglycemia could follow because, with no food absorption, the blood sugar remains perpetually low. So it seems the better part of wisdom to seek ways to overcome and heal this unpleasant problem. The following suggestions are the result of much research:

1) One tablespoon of psyllium powder or flakes dissolved in four ounces of distilled water, followed by a full glass of distilled water. (This has been given elsewhere for healing constipation also.)

2) Slippery elm herb capsule one to three times daily.

3) Add vitamin B6 to the diet.

4) One of the best natural aids for diarrhea is raw apple, which contains pectin. Even infants can safely be given the scrapings of a raw apple when suffering with loose bowels. Peel the apple and, with a spoon, scrape small bites from the apple. For some reason, this method aids better than eating the apple directly.

5) Garlic tablets or perles are very effective. Garlic is a natural healing substance known for its effectiveness in healing inflamed colons, and destroying bacteria which causes diarrhea.

6) Carob powder added to drinks is effective in healing diarrhea because of its high content of pectin, lignin, and all of the B vitamins. Pectin is found as a natural substance in the body. When the body experiences digestive difficulties it indicates pectin is in short supply. Foods containing pectin should form a large part of the diet to correct the problem. Carob powder is immediately effective in solidifying the stool. Purchase it at a health store. Mix it with raw whole milk for a delicious drink. Carob candy, minus the sugar and other undesirables, is also available from health stores. Carob is a substitute for chocolate. This is the most palatable "cure" imaginable since it is available in so many different forms.

7) A deficiency in the B vitamins results in diarrhea,

and a host of other ailments. So if diarrhea persists add foods high in B vitamins to your diet: apricots, beans, brewer's yeast, carrots, nuts, green leafy vegetables, whole grain cereals, wheat germ, soybeans, seeds. And take vitamin B in tincture form under the tongue for more direct absorption.

8) Diarrhea is a symptom of acute nicotine poisoning. So, smokers, if you experience persistent diarrhea your smoking could be the cause.

9) Try yogurt-prune whip as a snack. It will aid diarrhea, and also correct constipation. It certainly should be eaten during or after a course of antibiotics to restore destroyed beneficial bacteria.

10) Overdosing of vitamin D causes diarrhea. The usual intake is 1,000 milligrams daily, but see your doctor. Daily exposure to sunlight, which supplies vitamin D, should be before and after the five dangerous hours, which are between 10 a.m. and 3 p.m.

11) During a prolonged case of diarrhea don't restrict your salt intake. Diarrhea results in severe loss of salt. Make sure your source is vegetable or mineral salt. Purchase Real Salt or some other good brand from your health store. Or order mineral salt from the Dews Company (address elsewhere).

12) Drink raw vegetable juices. The pectin in the juices absorbs toxins and undesirable bacteria which may be causing the problem.

13) Are you regularly eating commercial ice cream? It could contain formaldehyde as well as many dyes and deadly chemicals. Such ice cream could cause not only diarrhea but a host of other problems. Instead choose ice cream with honey from your health store.

14) Potassium deficiency causes diarrhea. Avoid oral

diuretic drugs such as *Chlorothiazide*, which results in an excessive loss of moisture. Too frequent urination causes potassium depletion. Try juniper berries as a corrective herbal remedy. Also supplement the diet with potatoes, butter beans, navy beans, kale, dried peas, green leaf lettuce, parsnips, seafood from the deep sea, not the polluted shoreline type. Take potassium tablets or drink the apple cider vinegar-honey cocktail mentioned elsewhere.

15) Beware of "soft drinks" and sodas which contain, among other "things," artificial dyes, chemicals and sweeteners. The sweeteners are especially causative in diarrhea. Nursing mothers should especially avoid these beverages. They are often directly responsible for diarrhea and other drastic problems for their infants. Diarrhea in infants is a serious affliction. It could be fatal.

16) Drink raw buttermilk.

17) Eat ripe bananas and, again, apples. They both contain pectin, so needed to create soft bland stools that cleanse the intestines. The pectin also absorbs unfavorable bacteria and promotes the growth of favorable bacteria. Pectin can also be purchased in tablet form at your health store.

18) Be cautious in taking tryptophane, an amino acid tablet frequently lauded as an aid to nervousness and insomnia. Those allergic to it could develop diarrhea, splits around lips, sores on the tongue.

19) Be watchful for food allergies, especially pasteurized milk. Check your reaction to spices also.

20) Do eat much carrot soup. It not only contains many important nutrients, but it coats the inflamed intestines with a healing fluid. Also thick soup made with green beans and squash. Excellent! To make it more palatable, season with a vegetable bullion cube. Blend in

blender before serving, and add mineral salt and sesame oil when serving.

21) Take turmeric powder in capsules. It has proven remarkably effective.

22) In times of discomfort, choose the good standby Pepto Bismol over prescription drugs and other digestive "aids." It coats inflamed areas and absorbs acids which can cause distress.

Chapter Seven

The Urinary Tract

Elimination through the kidneys can usually be assured by drinking a sufficient quantity of water. If something additional is required, it is best to resort to herbs. Try usa urva. Watermelon seed tea or herb capsules are excellent, too, for flushing and purifying kidneys and bladder. Buchu tea or capsules are also excellent. A capsule combining all these herbs, plus juniper berries, parsley, goldenseal, ginger and Siberian ginseng bark, can be found at your health store. Drink apple cider or eat plenty of fresh apples.

Diuretics — Diuretics are water elimination pills given to treat such conditions as congestive heart failure. Their use can cause serious potassium depletion. A heart drug called *Digitalis* can also cause potassium loss. Patients taking *diuretics* regularly should also take a good source of potassium. Foods containing potassium include: tomatoes, oranges, dried apricots, cantaloupes, figs, raisins, bananas, prunes, sweet potatoes, potatoes and squash. A good source also is the apple cider vinegar-honey cocktail mentioned elsewhere.

Incontinence and Bladder Control — Incontinence is the loss of control of the sphincter muscle around the urethra. For continence, try the following remedy: 1/3 oz. of oak bark powder and one teaspoon of crushed juniper berries. Simmer for 5 minutes in 1/2 pint of water. Sweeten with honey. Take 3 tablespoons a.m. and p.m. Eat a lot of watermelon when in season. Or try cranberry capsules. They flush the bladder. They are excellent for treating incontinence. Once when I was experiencing a phase of incontinence, cranberry capsules corrected it. Don't take the kind with added sugar.

If these natural approaches aren't effective, there is a simple medical procedure which is an excellent alternative to conventional surgery. It's the injection of a paste and it has an almost one hundred percent record of correcting the problem. It's an in-office procedure that requires only a few hours. The paste is called GAX (Glutaraldehyde cross-linked collagen). GAX is a sterile injectable gel composed of a highly purified bovine dermal collagen that is cross-linked, increasing its stability. It is injected around the urethra. The collagen presses against the wall of the urethra, stopping the leakage of urine. It has been successful where even surgery has failed. Do inquire at any medical center to learn which doctors in your area are performing this simple procedure. Or see your gynecologist who can inquire. It's being done in various areas around the nation. Or have your gynecologist call Dr. Paul A. de Ridder in Santa Ana, California, who is specializing in this procedure and can refer you to a specialist in your area. Or consider a new simple procedure, called no-incision bladder suspension, now being performed. It requires only 30 minutes and only a two-day hospital stay. Have your doctor contact Dr. Sam Lipschitz, assistant clinical professor of surgery at Chicago Medical School or at Mt. Sinai Hospital Medical Center at Chicago.

Interstitial Cystitis or Bladder Disease — There is now a recognized treatment with dimethyl sulfoxide, better known as *DMSO*. If you suffer from this bladder disease and your doctor is not familiar with the treatments with DMSO, do have him contact the Cleveland Clinic in Cleveland, Ohio, for full information.

Kidney and Gallstones — Chocolate and oxalic food has been strongly linked to stones formed of calcium oxalate. All foods rich in oxalic acid help form kidney stones, and all other stones including gallstones. Stones may be a deficiency disease — a diet deficient in vitamins C and D, especially C. In areas of the world where vitamin C is lacking in the general diet, the population experiences kidney stones and bad teeth. Large doses of vitamin C usually clears cloudy urine and removes tartar from the teeth. Do eat foods rich in vitamin C such as citrus fruits, broccoli, mustard greens, green peppers, turnip greens, parsley, watercress, kale, Brussel sprouts and cabbage. In addition, take vitamin C supplements. You may see tartar deposits departing from your teeth which indicates similar deposits are departing from your entire system, thwarting the formation of stones or calcium deposits throughout the body.

Kidney stones can now be treated without anesthesia. The new treatment is called *second generation lithotripsy*. The treatment involves shock waves which are generated by using vibrating crystals. Anesthesia is not necessary, which makes the new treatment much safer than the treatment in the past, which was to dissolve the stones with electrical shock waves aimed at the kidneys. The shock waves were so powerful anesthesia was required. *Lithotripsy* requires less powerful shock waves. The patient lies on a table rather than in a tub of water. It's an out-patient procedure, requiring no more than two or three hours at a medical center.

The new method is extremely effective in dissolving painful kidney stones. The procedure may also be used to dissolve gallstones. If your doctor is not familiar with the procedure do have him contact Dr. Glen Preminger, assistant professor of Urology at the University of Texas in Dallas. A drug called *Thiola* is effective in halting the formation of cystine kidney stones, caused by an excess of the amino acid cystine. Also, see again the oil and whipping cream solution suggested in Chapter 5, as practiced by Dr. Som and as suggested by Jason Winters.

Incurable Kidney Disease — A drug is already available by prescription that is actually reversing a severe "incurable" kidney disease. It's call *Solu-Medrol*. It's been used for years to stop kidney transplant patients from rejecting their new organs. But now it's being used to eliminate the need for dialysis and kidney transplants. The severe form of kidney disease is known as RPGN (rapidly progressive glomerulonephritis). With Solu-Medrol the kidneys return to normal functioning and many patients are now avoiding the dialysis machine. The drug can be given at almost any major medical center.

For additional, up-to-date information regarding kidney disease there is a toll-free "hot line" number in the last chapter.

Chapter Eight

Reproductive System

Birth Control for Men? — In China doctors are experimenting with liquid polyurethane plastic injected into sperm ducts. It solidifies to act as a block, preventing the sperm from traveling to impregnate a female egg. Such use of plastic inside the human body may or may not have undesirable effects. Seems rather drastic to me. I don't see why the GAX collagen treatment for incontinence (see section on the Urinary Tract) couldn't also be effective in sealing the sperm ducts, just as it seals the area around the bladder to prevent urinary leakage. Just a thought. Researchers here in our country are finding that injections of a male hormone testosterone prevents sperm production, which resumes when the injections are stopped. This method of birth control is now being tested in many countries.

Birth Control Pills — Women taking the Pill as a contraceptive should be sure to eat green, leafy vegetables because they need a good source of folic acid.*

*See *Forever Young* , available at your bookstore or order from Astara.

Caesarean Births — Although in some instances a Caesarean section is absolutely necessary, Dr. Sidney M. Wolfe of the Public Citizen Health Research Group in Washington, DC, says many C-sections are needless. Dr. Wolfe points out that there are twice as many performed in the United States as elsewhere in the Western world. With today's technology — the sonagram, for instance — the opposite should be true. So, if you are pregnant and your doctor says a C-section is indicated, be sure to discuss it with him or her thoroughly — and don't be afraid to ask questions. Let them know of your total reluctance to submit to Caesarean surgery and agree to it only as a lifesaving necessity — because, ultimately, a C-section is far more open to major risks than vaginal delivery. Dr. Robert Cefalo, committee chairman, U.S. News & World Report, March 2, 1982, states that "up to 90,000 Caesarean sections could be avoided each year, considerably reducing the risk of maternal death, as well as length and cost of hospitalization."

Chlamydia — is a venereal disease which can now be detected with a new in-office test in less than 30 minutes. Chlamydia, left untreated, can cause abnormal pregnancies, pelvic inflammatory disease, birth defects, and infertility. The usual treatment is with the antibiotics tetracycline or erythromycin, both taken only as a last resort because of drastic side effects. Instead, contact Hanna Kroeger or Michael Tierra (see last chapter) to see if either offers herbal therapy for this infection.

Contraceptive Injections — There is now available a contraceptive drug called *Progestin* which can be given in the form of a shot every two or three months. It has been widely used in many other countries and has been just recently approved for use here in the United States.

Although it has a 99.7% rate of effectiveness, there could be side effects, such as difficulty conceiving after discontinuing the shots. So, if you are interested, discuss the possible side effects with your doctor.

Contraceptive Vaccine — Researchers at the University of Health Center in Farmington, Connecticut, report that an experimental contraceptive vaccine has blocked fertility without fail in both female and male guinea pigs. The vaccine's effect is temporary, fertility returning in the female in nine months, and in the male in seven months. Researcher Paul Primakoff cautions that many changes still must be developed before the vaccine could be seriously considered for humans.

Endometriosis — Infertility in women is usually caused by endometriosis. Endometriosis leads to the growth of uterine tissue outside a woman's uterus. It not only prevents conception but is the cause of considerable discomfort, even pain. A new laser treatment is now available, leaving women to become fertile again. The treatment takes about 30 minutes and the patient goes home that same day. If you are an infertile woman ask your doctor about *argon laser therapy* for endometriosis. It may be the answer to your problem of inability to conceive.

Hysterectomies — Dr. Franklin Loffer of St. Joseph's Hospital in Phoenix, Arizona, has pioneered a procedure involving a new infection-free laser technique which eliminates the need for a hysterectomy in women who suffer from excessive menstrual bleeding, to remove fibroid tumors (benign), and for patients who do not respond to hormonal therapy. The laser removes the uterus lining which causes the bleeding. It produces the same effect as the usual D&C (dilation and curettage). This procedure can be done without having to touch or cut the uterus. It's an out-patient procedure which can be performed in the doctor's office. It's half the price of conventional methods and requires only a couple of days to heal.

Also, Dr. Edward Marut at the University of Chicago, has been shrinking fibroid tumors of the uterus with injections of a drug called *Lupron*. He believes hysterectomies can often be avoided. Lupron shrinks the tumors so that they may be surgically removed without removing the uterus. It has some side effects. Do inquire of your doctor.

There is also a new type of laser surgery called *Rollerball*. It is now being used to avoid the usual drastic type of hysterectomy. If your doctor ever suggests hysterectomy, ask about this different approach.

Impotence — Impotence was once considered a psychological problem. But it is now recognized that most impotent men are suffering from an organic problem — usually poor blood circulation to the penis. It certainly is curable, and men should realize the cause is physical rather than psychological. It can be treated, just as high blood pressure or any other health problem can be treated. First of all, alcohol abuse is a leading culprit. It reduces the ability of the testicles to produce testosterone, a male hormone. Smoking is not only hazardous to your health but is disastrous to your sex life. It not only aids in contaminating the arteries, it significantly blocks the flow of blood in the reproductive glands, making erection impossible. Often these blocked arteries can be surgically opened, but it's not a lasting procedure unless the drinking/smoking habit is broken — along with a change in dietary habits. A low fat, high fiber diet is necessary to keep the arteries open.

There is now a new drug, *Phentolamine*, which dilates blood vessels and aids substantially in correcting impotence — but you may fare better with products from your health store than with drugs from your doctor. A reputed cure is an herb called *Yohimbine*, used as an aphrodisiac in Africa and Saudi Arabia for years. It was once jealously guarded in those countries but has now been made available worldwide as an herbal capsule. Yohimbine directly enlarges the blood vessels in the genital area. With the improved blood flow impotency disappears, especially if Yohimbine is combined with other herbs, such as Siberian ginseng or bee pollen.

The only problem is the Yohimbine plant is very delicate and blooms for only two weeks a year. Products containing Yohimbine, however, are available in many health stores and through mail order catalogs which sell health products (Swanson's for example). If you experience impotence or frigidity, be very sure your diet includes sufficient vitamins B and E.

See the section on cancer for information concerning testicle cancer. The new type of nerve-sparing surgery allows men to enjoy a normal sex life and father children, which wasn't possible with the conventional type of surgery.

Infertility — strikes far too many couples. In the female an ovulation problem, or blockages in the Fallopian tubes, is to blame. In the male, it is usually a low sperm count, which can be caused by stress, overwork, alcohol, tobacco, blocked arteries in the reproductive area. Couples experiencing infertility problems should contact the American Fertility Society or Resolve Inc. (See Chapter 20) They can refer you to physicians and scientists involved in research concerning infertility. There is now a procedure to clear blocked fallopian tubes, which is often the cause of infertility. It's the use of a balloon-tipped catheter to remove the blockages. The catheter is threaded into the blocked tube, the balloon is inflated, and the passage is cleared, allowing sperm and ovum to merge.

If you are trying unsuccessfully to become pregnant, you should stop drinking coffee. A new study at Maudsley Hospital in London shows that caffeine reduces fertility. The coffee stimulates the production of the hormone *prolactin* in women. Prolactin is known as "nature's own birth control."

Menopause — The process of the menopause is a perfectly normal happening but it creates many abnormal upsets. The ovaries slow their production of hormones, and often cease the production of estrogen altogether, leaving the adrenal-cortex to supply the estrogen needed by the body. Often the adrenal-cortex is not equipped to supply a sufficient production and the body suffers from a lack of estrogen. The most common abnormality is the hot flash which erupts like an inner volcano with a sudden surge of heat sweeping over the body, beginning at the face and neck. It's often accompanied by palpitations of the heart and a spacey feeling in the head.

Other abnormalities appear more slowly — wrinkles, double chins, gray hair, widening of the hips, increased waistline and osteoporosis or slowly bending spine. Ovulation, or the monthly menstrual flow, ceases — which means the ovaries no longer release the ovum-egg for possible fertilization. In some, the monthly period ceases gradually or it may cease suddenly without any preliminary warning.

The most common treatment is to place the patient on *estrogen therapy* together with *progesterone*. Many doctors fail to give the progesterone, not realizing how vital it is to the woman on estrogen therapy. Estrogen alone can create all manner of problems, including cancer of the cervix and breasts. Given with the progesterone, however, as nature meant it to be produced inside the body, will usually offset any problem the estrogen could cause. When estrogen ceases in the body, so does the natural production of progesterone. It makes no sense to replace the estrogen and not the progesterone.

If you are a candidate to receive estrogen therapy, be very sure to discuss with your doctor the wisdom of also receiving progesterone. Many physicians are aware that estrogen only becomes dangerous if it is not supplemented with the hormone progesterone. Without the progesterone to counterbalance the estrogen, estrogen can cause the uterus to over-produce tissue within the uterus and the cervix. Progesterone causes a sloughing off of these tissues, preventing the buildup of cancerous cells and tissues.

If your doctor decides to place you on estrogen replacement therapy but refuses to also place you on progesterone, do look for another doctor. Find one enlightened concerning a balanced estrogen-progesterone hormonal therapy. Also, ask for the lowest possible potency of estrogen. The lowest is a green tablet. The next lowest is the brown tablet. Ask for Premarin tablets. They are more natural than others. Their source is said to be from pregnant mares. Or ask for a tablet called *Estriol* instead of Premarin. It's from a more natural source. If your doctor isn't familiar with it, have him or her contact Dr. James Privitera at (818) 966-1618 for full information.

Many doctors place their patients simply on a vitamin E tablet which, for some, seems to be adequate to replace the lack of estrogen. The usual dosage is 400 IUs daily. If you have a history of high blood pressure, your doctor may wish to lower the intake or advise against the vitamin. But if you can take it, not only does the vitamin E therapy relieve hot flashes and other unpleasant symptoms, it also balances the blood pressure and relieves muscle pain. It reduces fatigue, nervousness and insomnia. It has been effective in patients experiencing severe or prolonged bleeding from the uterus. Vitamin E therapy is slow acting and results should not be expected for at least two or three months. If you are approaching the menopausal age, you would do well to make sure you get a good diet and that you take vitamin E daily. If so you may never experience the discomforts of menopause.

You might wish to couple it with the intake of G+, an herb tablet manufactured by Dynapro International, Inc. (address elsewhere) for the purpose of replacing estrogen therapy. G+ alone is sufficient for many who wish to avoid estrogen therapy. Coupling it with vitamin E could certainly be a wise substitute for estrogen.

Women experiencing the menopause may find kelp an aid in reducing the menopause symptoms, such as the hot flash. Women who take estrogen replacement therapy should also take nutritional safeguards against any negative effects. Some doctors suggest whole B complex vitamins, which detoxify the estrogen in the body. The best form of B complex is an under the tongue tincture, probably available at health stores. It's also available through Fanie, Inc.

There is also a new approach for women who cannot take estrogen replacement therapy by mouth or injection. It comes in the form of *Clonidine Skin Patches*, which seem effective in eliminating hot flashes. Discuss it with your doctor. The transparent, silver-dollar-sized skin patch releases estrogen through the skin. It reduces the risk of osteoporosis. It can be worn under clothing. A new patch is applied every three and a half days. The patch distributes estrogen in a similar way that it is naturally distributed. The hormone seeps directly into the bloodstream. Pills have to pass through the digestive tract and liver.

If you are the one out of five women who cannot use the patch because of skin irritation you soon will be able to take estrogen sublingually and still have the advantage of bypassing the stomach and liver. An added benefit is that the sublingual estrogen (under the tongue) is three to five times faster-acting than oral estrogen and has fewer side effects. Ask your doctor about it. Or Contact Dr. William Keye, professor of obstetrics and gynecology at the University of Utah.

Menstrual Cramps — If you suffer monthly pain you should eat more often and smaller portions during your "pain" days to maintain your blood sugar level. You should quickly discover which foods can trigger allergy headaches and avoid them. Keeping a daily food diary could be most helpful. You should also avoid alcohol before your period. You should eat foods rich in potassium, such as bananas, tomatoes and potatoes. There is now a tiny electric device which can be attached to the abdomen that relieves the pain through transcutaneous electrical nerve stimulation (TENS). The device can be worn under clothes.

Pain may also be avoided by adding vitamin E tablets to your diet, and wheat germ, or in taking extracted wheat juice. Pains during menstruation indicate a lack of vitamin B12 in the diet. Liquid vitamin B12 to be taken under the tongue may be ordered from Fanie International. (address elsewhere.) Delayed or irregular menstruation indicates a lack of sulfur. Try minute sulfur tablets known as Oxyquiniline. They can be obtained from Standard Homeopathic Pharmacy. (Address elsewhere) Or take an herbal capsule of Black Cohosh and your usual dosage of calcium. Or Dong Qui herb capsules. Elsewhere I've mentioned a product called G+. It too could be very helpful. It's an herb capsule. Apply a heating pad to the area also.

Miscarriage — Women who repeatedly lose their babies during pregnancy should know of a test showing an 85% success rate using low dosages of aspirin. One-fourth of an aspirin a day has proven highly effective. It's believed the aspirin promotes a healthy blood flow to the placenta and the fetus. Once pregnancy is determined, the mother-to-be should begin the aspirin therapy. Miscarriage occurs because of blood too thick to filter through to the fetus. Some pregnancies require a whole aspirin a day to thin the blood. Aspirin reduces the stickiness of thick blood and has been shown to be highly effective in avoiding miscarriage.

Pap Smears — Women who have experienced abnormal Pap smears have completely reversed the abnormality with the following treatment: alternating douches, perhaps two or three a week, using two tablespoons of *Glyco-thymoline* in a quart of warm water the first day, 15 drops of *Atomadine* in a quart of warm water the following day. Alternating these douches and applying a castor oil pack to the low abdomen for an hour a day brought about the reversal.

For further information concerning this treatment and for what is meant by "abnormal" Pap smears, do contact Doctors Gladys and William A. McGarey at the A.R.E. Clinic (address elsewhere). They habitually treat patients with Edgar Cayce remedies, of which Glyco-thymoline and Atomadine are two of the greatest. Order from Cayce Corner at the A.R.E. Clinic (address elsewhere). You may be interested in subscribing to their newsletter called *Pathways to Health*. If so, send an inquiry to them. Pathways contains many useful health ideas, usually all natural homeopathic or holistic. I think if I ever had a serious health problem, I'd head for their A.R.E. clinic in Phoenix, or to Hanna Kroeger in Boulder, Colorado.

So that you may be more familiar with Pap smear classifications: Class 1 is normal. Class 2 indicates slight abnormality, indicating inflammation but no malignancy. The inflammation could require treatment, after which the cervix returns to normalcy. Class 3 or 4 indicates a suspicion of malignancy. Class 5 indicates definite malignancy.

Virapap — is a new cervical cancer examination now available which gives more accurate results than the Pap smear. According to Dr. Richard Reid, of Wayne State University, in Detroit, *Virapap* detected eight more precancerous lesions than did the Pap smear.

Premenstrual Syndrome — can cause anguish and suffering to women each month just prior to menstruation. The pain can be caused by bacterial infections which can be easily cured. There are now two drugs which offer relief. One is *Mefenamic Acid*. The other is an antibiotic, *Doxycycline*. But this is only effective if the problem is caused by infection, not hormonal imbalances. You'll find further information in Chapter 9 under the heading of "PMS and the Thyroid."

Prostate — A balloon-tipped catheter is helping many men avoid prostate surgery. It's much like the type inserted in arteries to aid heart patients. This balloon unclogs the tubes that bring urine from the bladder. It also aids impotence, which can occur as a result of prostate surgery. It's similar to the balloon treatment described earlier to clear fallopian tubes in females.

Vaginal Dryness — Medical people call it *Dyspareunia*. It's not life threatening, but it can be uncomfortable and, in many cases, can prevent sex because of pain. Vaginal dryness is a natural part of life after 35, because the glands do not distribute as liberal a flow of estrogen as they once did. Estrogen regulates vaginal lubrication. When it fails to do so, vaginal tissues could become dry and painful. Other causes of such dryness are a lack of zinc, breast feeding an infant, oral contraceptives, stress, antidepressants, and some medications taken for heart problems and high blood pressure.

It usually first makes itself known by itching. It is often treated with an estrogen-progesterone therapy, prescribed by your doctor. Or it can be home-healed. Many use petroleum jelly (Vaseline) — I mention it because it's the *worst* possible approach to healing. It prevents the absorption of oxygen by vaginal tissues, increasing the problem. It can also cause infection. Petroleum jelly is a coal tar product — without all of the dangerous factions removed. So, although it may have other excellent uses, avoid Vaseline for this problem.

Instead, seek a non-prescription vaginal cream at your health store. There is one called *V-Aloe*, made with 70% Aloe Vera. There's another called *Perfect Match*, also containing Aloe Vera. Both are completely safe as natural lubricating gels. They restore the natural pH balance in the vaginal area. If not available, order from Swanson's. (address elsewhere.) Itching, however, can also be caused by candida albicans, a yeast infection. This problem may require a doctor's prescription. But do also contact Hanna Kroeger, who offers herbal remedies as a cure and preventive of candida. In any case, don't allow the itching to continue. Some causes can be quite serious. For further information concerning yeast infection, see Chapter 16. And see my book *Forever Young*.

Chapter Nine

The Thyroid and Thymus — Secret Centers of Youth

Thyroid — Dr. Lawrence Wood, president of the Thyroid Foundation of America in Boston, Massachusetts, states that one in every ten women suffer from an underactive thyroid, and that women are four times more likely than men to experience it. It is caused when the thyroid fails to produce a natural hormone called *Thyroxine*, which regulates body chemistry. It can be corrected by a prescription drug called *Synthroid*, which has many serious side effects — especially insomnia. So what can one do to correct the problem with natural methods?

Kelp is quite effective in the case of thyroid imbalances. It contains organic iodine. Each individual must experiment how much to take to be effective, usually one tablet daily. Take vitamin B6, too. Kelp is excellent for either an overactive or underactive thyroid, especially the hyper or overactive. Usually the victim will be thin and nervous.

For the hypo or underactive thyroid victim — the overweight type — kelp in tincture is advisable, if obtainable.

Also, ask your doctor about taking potassium gluconate or diuretic herbs to control fluids until the thyroid gland normalizes. A tiny bar magnet may be advisable. Place the north pole of the magnet against the Adam's apple near the thyroid to correct an underactive thyroid. Place the south pole against the gland to correct one that is overactive. Hold it in place with a beauty chin strap or any kind of elastic bandage. Communicate with Bio Health Enterprises, Inc. (address elsewhere) for ordering bar magnets and to get further information. They also sell a product called *T-100*, an organic iodine product.

An Overactive Thyroid — will produce feelings of being sweaty and hot, unexplained weight loss, weakness in muscles such as trouble climbing stairs, hands that shake, rapid pulse, breast pain, bulging eyes, irregular menstrual periods. Try the south pole of a bar magnet over the thyroid gland.

An Underactive Thyroid — Those with an underactive thyroid often experience panic attacks. If you suffer from panic attacks, which are activated stress, do have your doctor check for any type of thyroid problem. Low thyroid, or hypothyroidism, can cause low energy, undue fatigue, repeated infections, headaches, circulatory disturbances and menstrual difficulties. It can also be a culprit in heart attacks. For further information, see Chapter 10 concerning *Heart Attacks and the Thyroid.* It may also be connected with muscle aches and weaknesses, some hearing disturbances, memory loss and concentration difficulties, cold hands and feet, thinning hair. There may be neuralgic pain. Another effect could be eczema and other skin problems such as psoriasis. Acne patients may also benefit from thyroid treatment. Chronic boils and one infection after another have been caused by thyroid deficiency. Repeated miscarriages may also be a result. In such cases the thyroid often has become too alkaline — try the cider vinegar-honey cocktail described elsewhere. The hydrogen ion is too low. Try also the north pole of a bar magnet over the thyroid. Or try homeopathic remedy *N-14*. Standard thyroid tests often fail to detect the problem.

Major warning signs to indicate an underactive thyroid are general fatigue, weight gain without increased eating, constipation, swollen face, brittle fingernails and hair, leg cramps, sore muscles, dry rough skin, longer and heavier periods each month.

The following symptoms may be present with either an overactive or underactive thyroid: premature gray hair, rheumatoid arthritis, patchy hair loss, white spots on the skin, a family history of diabetes or thyroid problems. Try practicing the thyroid therapy offered in the book *Forever Young* to stimulate the thyroid to restore youthful vigor and encourage the endocrine system to balance its hormonal flow. It's an acupressure procedure. Or try some of the other natural treatments listed in this chapter. Or write Swanson's for suggested thyroid therapy (natural approach) in order to avoid prescription drug therapy. However, be sure to see your doctor if you experience any problems.

The Thyroid and PMS (Premenstrual Syndrome) — Ninety-four percent of premenstrual syndrome women tested in a study were found to be deficient in thyroid hormones. If you suffer from PMS and would like to discover if you, too, are deficient, there is a home method of discovery. Take your underarm temperature for ten minutes before getting out of bed in the morning. If your temperature is consistently below 97.8, you probably have an underactive thyroid and should ask your doctor to prescribe thyroid medication. Or try the north pole of a bar magnet. Or kelp.

The Thymus and the Crystal Laser — Hanna Kroeger has just produced a *crystal laser* device which stimulates the thymus and the vibration of the spinal fluid. It looks much like a flashlight with a large head. It contains a conditioned laser beam which, directed toward the thymus gland, strengthens the immune system, aids in preventing colds, flu, viral infections and increases a positive attitude. The special golden crystals and the special herbs inside the device emit life energy and orgone energy. Its laser ray projects a magenta color, which is the healing color for the thymus gland and the immune system. Hanna claims it is of Atlantean origin. Contact her personally for full information. It is strongly suspected that the thyroid and thymus are directly connected with the aging process — and with proper stimulation and hormonal balance could contribute unquestionably toward retaining youth.

Chapter Ten

Attacking the Heart Attack

In the early years of the twentieth century, heart attack was a very rare occurrence. The great heart specialist, Dr. Paul Dudley White, stated that when he graduated from medical college in 1911 he had never seen or heard of a case of coronary occlusion. What has happened in 80 years to have brought it to epidemic proportions? In those early days, our foreparents mostly ate fresh garden vegetables and fresh butchered meats. Certainly their foods were not saturated with all manner of preservatives, chemical sprays, antibiotics and artificial hormones. And their dairy products were not so pasteurized as they are today. Their eggs came from "ground free" chickens, their breads were whole wheat products mostly baked at home. Their salt was mined with full spectrum minerals. What a difference in the diet of today!

I'm sure your dentist has told you about "plaque" forming on the teeth and the importance of flossing to remove the plaque daily. But what about the "plaque" that forms on the linings of the coronary arteries? Like plaque on teeth, it's of a consistency of toothpaste which eventually hardens. It's called arteriosclerosis or hardening of the arteries.

Through the years this sludge builds up so that blood has great difficulty in reaching the heart through these hardened arteries. The coronary or heart arteries are occluded, which means they are "closed off." When a patient suffers what his physician calls a *coronary occlusion*, it means the blood has not been able to reach the heart. It can mean instant death. If the patient survives, the doctor usually prescribes an anticoagulating drug to prevent blood from clotting and adding additional occlusion to coronary arteries. These drugs are manmade, of chemicals that thin the blood but also produce side effects. Aspirin will also thin the blood with few side effects.

When a blood clot breaks away from a wound in the intestinal lining of the stomach and floats on the bloodstream through too narrow a channel on its way to the heart, it may block an artery altogether, causing a heart attack. Such an attack is called *thrombosis*. The clot moving along the bloodstream is called an *embolus*.

As the bloodstream becomes increasingly sluggish and the coronary arteries leading to the heart muscle become increasingly hardened with toxic debris, it causes a decrease in the blood supply reaching the heart muscle. This is what causes the severe chest pains known as *angina pectoris*.

Angina heart attacks occur when the heart has been forced to labor constantly to pump blood through narrowed arteries until the heart is simply fatigued. When arteries are obstructed with hardened waste matter, urea or uric acid builds up in the system, creating a hardship on an overworked heart. That is when the angina heart attack occurs. The urea is a result of undigested protein. The buildup of this rotting waste material in arteries causes the heart to overwork and the colon to become obstructed through constipation.

The allopathic doctor, seeking to eliminate the problem, first thinks of a drug to thin the blood. Or he may suggest you immediately submit to surgery to remove the hardened plaque from the arteries. He may suggest an angioplasty procedure which injects a substance into the blood vessels to determine the major seat of your problem — so that bypass surgery can be more successfully performed. But seldom will he focus on major changes in the diet. The holistic doctor will immediately think of chelation therapy, which points toward avoiding surgery.* Such a procedure certainly requires major dietary changes. Both will probably think of reducing cholesterol, but their approaches may differ widely.

Any type of heart problem is the result not only of undigested protein but too much refined white salt, too much refined white sugar, too much refined white flour in the system. *The body itself then begins to produce an overabundance of cholesterol to fight the salt-sugar-paste buildup.* It is then that cholesterol becomes dangerous. Your own body produces cholesterol as the body's own natural defense, because the subconscious knows cholesterol is required to help blood pass through the arteries. The subconscious recognizes the white sugar, salt, flour as foreign substances invading the body and seeks to protect the arterial system from such an invasion by releasing its own cholesterol.

*See *The Book of Beginning Again.*

But such a cholesterol buildup dilates arteries and veins. And when arteries and veins are coated with hardened waste debris, they lose their flexibility — their ability to expand and contract. When this happens breaks and wounds occur along the arteries and veins. A blood clotting substance rushes to the wound in an attempt to heal. An angina heart attack may occur when some of the clotting is released in the bloodstream or fragments of cholesterol float on the bloodstream.

Either of these clots floating on the bloodstream could plug a heart valve, causing it to go into spasm. If the blood clot or the cholesterol cannot be dissolved, the blood builds up around the heart. If the buildup becomes severe enough, arteries or veins could burst around the heart, causing an angina attack.

Hardened Arteries — sludge in the arteries — has only come about since we began eating refined white flour, refined white sugar and refined table salt. That's why Dr. Paul Dudley White never heard of a case of coronary occlusion in his day. Our diet didn't include refined white flour, sugar and salt in those days. *Refined white flour* is wheat grain with the germ and all the natural health-giving properties removed, leaving only a white powdery substance called "pure improved refined flour." Mixed with milk or water in bread or pastry making, it becomes "pure paste" in the system, eventually packing down into sludge, plaque, and hardened substance. . . much like plaque on the teeth.

Hardly anyone is not acquainted with the cholesterol-heart attack controversy. The first thing your allopathic doctor will do if a heart attack threatens is to remove eggs from your diet and advise you to consume polyunsaturated fats. But he usually says not a word about tossing away your *refined white sugar.* He sees no connection between refined white sugar and heart attack. Yet, naturopaths and psychic healers involved in turning us towards a natural diet have long been warning that one of the principal culprits in heart attack is white sugar. The human body is incapable of absorbing or digesting inorganic substances. They crystallize in the joints and body tissues, hardening arteries and impeding blood circulation. Inorganic sodium chloride, or *salt*, is another of the worst offenders. You must eat salt in its organic form — a mineral salt.

So there you have again the three deadly whites which the body rejects as foreign substances. When there is a constant invasion of white salt, sugar and white flour, the body, releasing its own supply of cholesterol in an effort to destroy this foreign matter, creates a buildup of too much cholesterol. It is seldom due to eating too many eggs, which is the usual assumption. *It is caused because the body produces increased cholesterol in an effort to rid the body of processed salt, sugar and white flour.*

White sugar is utterly lacking in essential vitamins, minerals, amino acids, and essential fatty acids. It's a "dead" food. To consume it is to substitute it for foods which the body needs. White sugar leaches vitamins and minerals from the body's reserves so the body can utilize the sugar, leading to all manner of diseases, such as diabetes, hypoglycemia, high blood pressure and, assuredly, heart problems.

Add wheat germ to your diet (unless you are allergic to wheat). It has its own inbuilt anticoagulant substance that prevents blood from clotting and keeps it thin. It should become part of your diet long before you ever suffer a heart attack. But if you are already having heart difficulties, certainly it should become a part of your daily diet. It is nature's anticoagulant "medicine" and results in no harmful side effects whatsoever. Take a spoonful daily. This reinforces the idea that removing the germ from wheat to make white flour (white bread) is a major cause of heart problems caused by blocked arteries. Putting wheat germ back in your diet is essential.

Refined white salt crystallizes in arteries and in joints. *A rapid rise in cholesterol is the body's own way of destroying its enemy — refined salt*. Salt is only good when it is combined with all the other natural minerals — such as Real Salt from your health store. Or you can order it from Canyon's, (see last chapter) if your health store doesn't carry it. Or order mineral salt from the Dews Company.

Heart Attacks and the Thyroid — Dr. Broda O. Barnes, a thyroid specialist in Fort Collins, Colorado, has written a book titled, *Solved — the Riddle of Heart Attacks.* He vigorously asserts that cholesterol is not the culprit behind the heart attack disaster. To him, research has proven that a low cholesterol diet does nothing to prevent arteries from hardening and it is hardening arteries that causes heart attacks.

His theory is that a malfunctioning thyroid gland causes hardening of the arteries which lead directly to heart attack. (But what causes the malfunctioning thyroid? — couldn't it be a wrong diet?) His 50 years of research and practical practice has discovered that thyroid therapy corrects elevated blood serum fats and cholesterol. His patients, who have been on thyroid therapy for years, very rarely suffer a heart attack. He declares that hardening of the arteries results from thyroid deficiency, not from elevated serum fats that accompany it. In his book Dr. Barnes offers a no-cost method for checking whether or not you have a thyroid deficiency.

To repeat, shake down a thermometer and place it near at bedtime. When you waken in the morning place it snugly under an armpit for ten minutes. The normal range of temperature is 97.8 to 98.2 Fahrenheit. If you persistently get a low reading it could possibly indicate you need thyroid therapy. Dr. Barnes states that the medical profession has been reluctant to accept what he calls this basal temperature test. He explains that it is too simple and that no money can be made from it. Also, many physicians resent patients trying to make a diagnosis on themselves. But he has spent fifty years developing his theory and, in his book, indicates he has saved many lives. So why not test yourself to discover whether or not you have a low temperature reading? If so, consult your doctor about thyroid therapy. Or take kelp tablets.

Dr. Barnes states that thyroid therapy raises the metabolism and because of this, more B vitamins are required. He suggests brewer's yeast tablets. Since Dr. Barnes is a thyroid specialist, many of his patients are naturally seeking help with a thyroid problem. They are placed on small doses of thyroid, usually an initial dosage of 1/2 grain daily. After one or two months, the dosage is increased 1/2 grain at a time and, in some cases, over a period of six months, increased to 2 grains daily.

With this therapy he has helped those who have had heart attacks return to a normal life. He has saved many others from potential heart attacks, in that the great percentage of his patients simply never develop either hardening of the arteries or experience a heart attack. This report of his researches is included here because he may be right. Do purchase his book and decide for yourself. Reading it could save your life. See again my chapter concerning the thyroid, the thymus and keeping young.

Heart Attack and the Diet — It's possible the buildup of thyroid hormones could overcome the effects of a bad diet — because *an overabundance of cholesterol will suppress the function of the thyroid.* Now if the overabundance of natural cholesterol has been created because the body itself is attempting to overcome the effect of too much salt, sugar, and white flour, then the basic cause of the problem is not the builtup cholesterol, not a deficient thyroid, but too much refined "whites." *It is recognized that elevated cholesterol can be brought under control with thyroid therapy.* So while you are testing for a thyroid deficiency, and taking thyroid therapy to offset the deficiency, do give thought to a change in diet.

Since Pritikin proved diet is very much involved in heart and artery problems, it would appear that the way to avoid problems is to look to the diet in the first place — not only for heart problems but just to maintain good health. Anyway, let me share my ingathered research with you concerning this major health problem. Let's begin with Dr. Som, the naturopath who taught me so much about natural methods of healing, and whose teachings were echoed in my book *Beginning Again.* He first taught me how to switch from white sugar, white salt, white flour:

For refined white sugar he suggested substituting date sugar. Or white sugar from vegetables, with all the good elements left in. He used a lot of raw honey. He used maple sugar. For refined white salt, he substituted a product called Real Salt, it's mineral salt, which is salt with all the other minerals with it. Instead of refined white flour he always used whole wheat products or rye.

(I repeat, all through this book, I'll be telling you the names of various products and the distributor, but I'll say "address elsewhere." That means you'll find the address in the last chapter.)

Dr. Som surprised me when he said the diet should include arsenic. After recovering from my shock, he added that some foods, such as asparagus and celery, contain minute particles of arsenic which, in this natural form, is excellent for the heart. He called them "homeopathic foods" and he called God the Supreme Homeopath. He said a couple of cayenne herb capsules with a cup of warm water could stop a heart attack. He suggested making cayenne herb capsules part of your daily vitamin therapy. Taking plenty of brewer's yeast flakes or tablets daily relieves much of the pain in heart disease. It contains biotin and it's the action of the biotin which relaxes muscular contractions around the heart. If yeast causes gas problems, try adding a bit of lemon juice to the water with which you swallow the yeast.

Dr. Som agreed that polyunsaturated cold pressed fats were to be chosen over saturated processed animal fat. But even they should not be used liberally, especially in cooking. It is far better to add the oils to food when it is served as a substitute for butter. Unsaturated fats should never be oxidized by heat in cooking. Such heat produces extremely toxic lipid peroxides. Consuming heated oil transforms normal cells into ceroid pigments and the accumulative effect of this cell destruction is premature aging. Cooking unsaturates causes them to form polymers, a chemical compound similar to plastics, varnish and shellac which, taken into the body, increases toxicity.

This is one reason fried foods are to be strictly avoided, especially in a restaurant. Those "delicious" French fries have no doubt been fried in stale restaurant grease that has been repeatedly heated hour after hour. Such an intake of toxic heated oil is disastrous to the body. This is why you must choose unrefined cold-pressed oils.

Oils processed the usual way could involve the use of petroleum products that could retain toxic insecticide residues, or heated animal fats. Processed oils, solidified fats and "lard" usually contain the preservatives BHT and BHA which have been implicated in birth defects and brain damage — and are certainly responsible for increasing the level of cholesterol.

Many people now resort to eating "cholesterol-free" imitation egg substitutes, proudly believing they are protecting the body from the dreaded cholesterol. Beware! They do very little to lower the cholesterol level, but they load your body with a chemical preservative which your own natural cholesterol rises to attack as a foreign substance.

Doctors often prescribe a cholesterol-lowering drug called *Clofibrate*. They do so knowing that the drug has been linked with blood clots, heart pain, irregular heart beat and gallstones. Niacin is also frequently prescribed in megadoses to lower cholesterol. But taken in such massive doses, it can cause gastrointestinal problems, abnormalities in heart rhythms, and disturbances in body chemistry. It should be taken only in moderate dosages. So said Dr. Som.

Dr. Som constantly warned about drinking pasteurized or homogenized milk. It not only aids in heart attacks but it also is a culprit in arthritis. So if you must drink milk, try to obtain raw certified whole milk. Dr. Som called homogenized milk, or even low fat milk, a "fractured" food. He said separating the milk from the cream, or processing the milk so that the fat of the cream is evenly distributed throughout the milk — which is homogenization — caused the milk to be harmful.

Now comes a report from Dr. Oster, chief of cardiology

at Park City Hospital in Bridgeport, Connecticut, to substantiate what Dr. Som tried so hard to tell his patients to prevent them from suffering heart attacks. Dr. Oster says: "Homogenized milk (the common form sold throughout America) is a major cause of heart disease in the U.S." He says the fat in the milk contains a substance called *xanthine oxidase*, or XO, an enzyme which will enter the bloodstream once the milk is homogenized. The XO acts chemically to scar the walls of the arteries. The body's own defense system acts to repair the damage by raising the level of cholesterol in the blood, and depositing protective fatty material to heal the scars. "When the old-fashioned non-homogenized milk is drunk," he says, "the body excretes the XO like any other waste." He says if one habitually drinks homogenized milk, the fatty material in the blood begins to obstruct the arteries, causing heart problems.

Dr. Kurt Esselbacher, chairman of the Department of Medicine at Harvard Medical School, agrees. So does Dr. Donald J. Ross, professor of biology at Fairfield College, Connecticut. Dr. R. Lincoln Kessler, chief attending physician at Rush-Presbyterian St. Luke Medical Center, says the first thing he does with heart patients is to take them off homogenized milk.

The patients who are given folic acid (a B vitamin), and ascorbic acid (vitamin C), both of which combat the action of XO, experience dramatic results, says Dr. Oster. He claims the damage is begun in early childhood, when children are encouraged to drink a lot of milk. They should be drinking only raw whole milk — or none at all.

In addition to adding wheat germ to the diet, Dr. Som prescribed a daily tablet of vitamin E containing from 200 to 400 International Units. These tablets, the wheat germ itself, or a spoonful of wheat germ oil will contain the natural anticlotting substance that our grandparents received in their home-baked natural wheat bread and pastries, before white bread emerged on the scene. Many physicians, agreeing with Dr. Som, will temporarily place their heart patients on much larger dosages, ranging from 1600 to 2400 units of vitamin E a day. Research reveals that this increased dosage will dissolve coronary scars, reverse electrocardiographic abnormalities, and dissolve blood clots. It's an aid to protecting the lungs from air pollution.

Dr. Julian Whitaker, author of *Reversing Heart Disease*, warns against indiscriminate bypass surgery. Having treated over 3000 heart patients, he has found the most effective treatment to be fresh farm produce, walking or running and regular exercise. He suggests 3 meatless meals a week, fresh green salads twice a day, at least one fresh fruit daily, and oat bran in your daily diet. He says there's no guarantee you'll survive bypass surgery and there's a very good chance you'll suffer brain damage if you do.

Dr. Som insisted on some measure of exercise daily and regularly. This is extremely important for prevention or for the cardiac patients. They cannot become sedentary, they must remain active. Try moderately rapid walking. Or walking up and down stairs. Climb steep hills. Walk on sand at the beach. Lie on the floor with the feet in the air riding an imaginary bicycle. Or lie on a slant board and pedal in the air for greater benefit. Or buy a stationary bicycle. The exercise need not be vigorous but it certainly should be regular. One is forced to breathe deeply which brings oxygen into the lungs and burns up waste matter. Dr. Som said to regain health after a heart attack, focus on exercise, not excessive rest.

Dr. Som was totally opposed to coffee. He said coffee

was a culprit in heart attacks. Research discloses that more than five cups a day results in twice the risk of severe coronary disease as those drinking no coffee at all. But Dr. Som said that caffeine in even one cup would cause a rise in blood pressure which could last up to 45 minutes — and could imbalance the endocrine glands for hours. If one is under stress caffeine could increase the stress. He said coffee residue in the system settled around bicuspid valves in the veins, which prevented the free flow of blood. Even if the arteries weren't clogged, if these valves were sluggish in opening, the blood circulation was very poor. He prescribed homeopathic remedies but I don't remember what they were. However, since then I've found remedies which are credited with cleaning the sludge from the arteries and some which remove the residue around valves in the veins.

Hanna Kroeger sells an herbal product called *Circu-Flow* which, taken with aloe vera gel three times a day, will act as oral chelation therapy. (Address elsewhere). See my *Book of Beginning Again* for my own experience with chelation. Hanna's herbal remedy includes Equisetum Concentrate, Hawthorne berries and Quaw Bark. She says that, taken as directed, even one bottle will go far toward clearing out the sludge. She says the formula was given her by a Higher Source. Michael Tierra offers an herbal remedy right out of the rain forests of Brazil. He's a reborn modern Medicine Man whose knowledge of herbal therapy surpasses anyone I know — and his herbs come from far away lands where herbs have long been known to heal every illness mankind experiences.

I've heard, too, of a product called *Rodaquin*, supposed to be effective in rejuvenating the vascular system. It's a new cellular nutrient said to be totally natural, not a drug. For further information, write to Rodaquin Laboratories.

(Address in last chapter.) Dynapro International sells an herbal product called *AR+* which not only removes plaque from arteries but also the deposits around the vein valves. (Address elsewhere.) Both are excellent products.

Dr. Som insisted on including garlic in the diet in some form, even taken in odorless capsules if necessary. It has proven effective against a high cholesterol level, lowering it drastically. It is also effective as a natural antibiotic. Its healing properties are effective in healing breaks and injuries in the artery walls and in killing low grade intestinal infections. He advocated folic acid, which performs wonders against hardening of the arteries.

He suggested a raw food diet for a while, or raw salads with just a bit of cooked foods added, along with wheat breads, date sugar and vegetable salt. He insisted on wheat germ oil or flaxseed oil added to breakfast juices. Or a tablespoon of flaxseed swallowed down with water, which not only cleaned sludge from the arteries but started natural bowel movements to remove wastes from impacted colons. The flaxseed can be ground in a nut grinder if you prefer.

He advocated amino acids. He said an amino acid called *carnitine* could prevent a buildup of blood around the heart, which caused the excruciating pain of angina. Since then, tests conducted at the University of Wisconsin have vindicated him. Carnitine, an amino acid, is found naturally in a healthy heart. Given as medication against a heart attack, it has none of the serious side effects usually associated with conventional angina drugs. Carnitine causes the heart to utilize fats in the cells instead of sugars.

Dr. Som was strong on adding lecithin to the diet, available from the health store. It has proven effective against high levels of cholesterol and in protecting the body against hardening of the arteries. He said that with the development of arteriosclerosis, the brain is apt to be the first to suffer a lack of blood flow. So he suggested exercises to nourish the brain — to help the blood reach the brain:

Lie face down on the bed with the head hanging over the edge. Just this simple act provides a traction to the neck, allowing blood to flow freely to the brain. Let your head hang thusly for at least five minutes. Repeat it twice a day. If you do not seem to obtain enough of a head hang, then assume the knee-chest position with the knees and chest on the edge of the bed. With the head hanging over the side of the bed in this fashion, the traction in the neck is increased even more. Lie in this position from five to fifteen minutes. To increase the benefits during the traction, perform the "Breath of Fire," (panting with the lips closed). If the Breath of Fire is uncomfortable then simply perform long, slow, deep inhalations and exhalations.

Dr. Som, ever alert to heal through natural means, pointed to carob as a means of preventing heart attacks. He knew it had been used by the ancient Greeks to heal diarrhea. He sometimes called it the locust bean and said this was the locust of Biblical fame, eaten by John the Baptist in the desert. He said the gum of the bean was total fiber which would reduce the damage created by cholesterol and other fats. The gum of the carob bean is almost identical to guar gum, which is a recognized enemy of cholesterol.

Dr. Som said if one should have a heart attack while alone, while waiting for help to arrive one should cough deep down coughs, with deep breaths between and continue until help arrives. Deep breaths flood the lungs while the coughing pumps the heart and keeps blood circulating. He also immediately prescribed vitamin B6 for the heart patient. He said B6 attacked undesirable elements in the blood.

Choose unrefined sesame seed oil, canola or olive oil for your kitchen use. Make your salad dressing of these oils, which are rich in vitamin E. Put them in your soup when you serve it, eat them with your baked potatoes instead of butter, eat over your steamed vegetables — such as greens, asparagus or artichoke — rather than butter.

He always demanded a reduction of protein in the diet. He said Americans ate far too much daily. He said this could explain the cause of mysterious crib deaths among infants — a buildup of too much protein in the infant body, caused by cow's milk. Cow's milk cannot be properly digested by an infant. Undigested protein becomes urea in the system. When the system becomes overloaded with urea, the infant's heart simply cannot handle the overload and a heart attack snuffs out its life. He prescribed a soy milk formula if mother's milk is too scarce.

He advocated fiber to avoid heart attacks. He often suggested steel cut oatmeal. He cooked it with raisins. He used blackstrap molasses or date sugar as a sweetener. He added Mocha Mix instead of cow's milk. He also suggested oat bran and whole grain bread. Hippocrates, whose oath is still followed by all physicians, highly recommended that his patients eat whole meal bread for its "salutary effects on the bowels." So do add whole meal bread containing oat bran if you can find it. Oat bran and all fiber foods are recognized as a means of improving elimination. This indirectly prevents constipation and diverticulitis.

Fiber is even recognized as a means of healing ulcers, even though it is "roughage." Fiber, the indigestible part of the foods we eat, consists of the bran in grains and the pulp in fruit and fibrous vegetables. Fiber consists of five basic forms: pectin, gum, lignin, cellulose, and hemicellulose. Pectin and gums, working chemically, prevent the absorption of undesirable substances into the bloodstream, such as fats. Oat bran is a source of water-soluble fiber containing a gum called veta-glucan. Cellulose, lignin and hemicellulose act as sponges. They absorb water and expand in the intestines, creating a "full" feeling and reducing the appetite. They also soften stools, which prevents constipation. Dr. Som said that a drop in blood pressure could be obtained even by taking a fiber tablet daily, though he much preferred food roughage. He sent his patients to the health store to purchase activated charcoal tablets, because he said it not only reduced flatulence but lowered cholesterol in the blood.

He was persistent about potassium. He said it protected against high blood pressure and lowered the risk of a stroke. He started all his patients on the apple cider vinegar-raw honey cocktail, but only once a day. He emphasized fruits with potassium, such as bananas, oranges, grapefruit. Being a vegetarian, he ate a lot of potatoes, loaded with natural potassium. He said potassium foods prevented high blood pressure from damaging cells which line the arteries, although they didn't actually lower blood pressure. They just prevented artery damage.

He highly endorsed the breakfast I've eaten for years — fresh orange juice blended with a teaspoon each of lecithin granules, yeast flakes, goat milk whey powder, mixed seeds with dried apple and banana flakes, one teaspoon of flaxseed, one tablespoon of flaxseed oil and one of liquid chlorophyll. (If interested, order some of these from Arthur Blackmer, address elsewhere.) Or purchase from health stores. I eat this enriched orange juice with five freshly shelled almonds daily. Occasionally I eat six prunes soaked overnight. And I drink one cup of vinegar-honey cocktail. This breakfast gives me hours of unbounded energy.

During his lectures, Dr. Som never tired telling of the miraculous power of the onion. I've heard him say it would counteract the effects of fat in the diet. Now comes a report to vindicate him. Eating onions with a high-fat meal may reduce the chances of a heart attack or stroke, suggests Dr. A. S. Truswell of Queen Elizabeth College:

"We found after a fat meal the (blood) platelets stuck together faster than the platelets of the subjects who had eaten the ordinary meal. But when onion was included in the high fat meal, this effect was neutralized. It's really amazing. Platelets are a component in the blood concerned with stopping bleeding. When their function goes wrong, they form clots which are involved in thrombosis in arteries to the brain and heart...resulting in heart attacks and strokes. Onions tend to decrease the clotting power of blood."

Dr. Som said that taking garlic tablets after such a meal would too.

A report on the benefits of diet states that one tablespoon of olive oil cancels out the cholesterol effect of two eggs. Cholesterol is also lowered by eating two apples a day; or a cup of dried beans; or two raw carrots; or two grapefruit; or four ounces of oat bran. And raw onion should be eaten daily. (Take a salute Dr. Som.)

To really clean the arteries, not only should the diet be changed, but one must exercise, reduce stress and give up smoking. To prevent a second heart attack many doctors prescribe *beta blockers* — which help control irregular heartbeats by preventing the hormone adrenaline from reaching the heart.

Home cholesterol tests enable you to check your own levels. The home kit contains a needle used to prick a finger and a chemically treated card which contains a color-coded chart. Matching your blood droplet tells you if your cholesterol level is high, low, borderline or satisfactory. Normally, a reading above 240 is high, 200-239 in borderline, below 200 is satisfactory. Do remember that home tests of any kind should not replace tests by a trained physician.

Heart Disease and Aspirin — Some doctors recommend taking an aspirin every other day, which has been known to cut the risk of heart attacks by nearly 50%. Some suggest a fourth of an aspirin daily. Others suggest two aspirin daily. Without a doubt, the intake of aspirin can affect the vascular system. It acts as a blood thinner, thus preventing strokes. There is no reason not to take some aspirin therapy if one is a candidate for heart disease, but one cannot rely totally upon such an approach. The diet absolutely must be considered as a major means of not only preventing heart disease but as a secondary means of prolonging youth, beauty and health.

One also cannot ignore the findings that vitamins C and E inhibit buildup of cholesterol deposits in artery walls. Vitamin E also interferes with blood clotting, an aid to preventing strokes. If you take aspirin daily, as do many heart patients and arthritics, do also take increased amounts of vitamin C — from 2000 to 6000 mgs. a day. The aspirin leaches vitamin C from your system. But remember, if you stop the aspirin therapy for any reason, don't stop the intake of vitamin C immediately. Slowly reduce the daily dosage.

Irregular Heartbeat — Surprise! If you've been apprehensive because of irregular or "chaotic" heartbeat, stop worrying. Harvard Medical School researcher Ary Goldberber has reported to the American Association for the Advancement of Science that an irregular heartbeat is actually the sign of a healthy heart. A normal heartbeat fluctuates over any given time period, he says, but steadies into a wavelike consistent beat just prior to a sudden heart failure. Lordy, Lordy! — who is right!? Seems we're "doomed" if it do, and "doomed" if it don't!

High Blood Pressure — If you have high blood pressure, avoid licorice in any form. It aggravates high blood pressure or can counteract the effectiveness of medication for the problem. If you're taking drugs prescribed for depression or high blood pressure you should avoid such foods as aged cheese, chianti wine and chicken livers. (Well, who wants to eat chicken livers, anyway. Probably contributed to high blood pressure in the first place!) The drugs given can react with a substance called *pyramine*, an amino acid in these foods, which would force the blood pressure to dangerous levels, resulting even in death.

Such patients should also avoid pickled herring, fermented sausages, salami, pepperoni, sharp cheeses, yogurt, sour cream, beef and chicken livers, broad beans, canned figs, bananas, avocados, soy sauce, active yeast preparations, beer, sherry and other wines in large quantities, cola beverages, coffee, chocolate and raisins. Nor should such a patient consume alcohol. Well, like I said — eating can be hazardous to your health!

If your doctor has prescribed the drug *Hydralazine* it can deplete the body of vitamin B6, so if you take this drug, take the entire family of B vitamins, emphasizing B6. A new drug called *Cartrol* is being used to lower blood pressure. Fiber supplements also lower blood pressure. And cholesterol levels. After exercising, don't take your pulse at the neck. Pressure on the carotid artery could slow the heart rate too much too quickly.

Chocolate contains a chemical called *phenylethylamine* that affects the brain by releasing sudden bursts of energy. This chemical works by constricting blood vessels and raising blood pressure. This chemical in chocolate is also responsible for migraine headaches. So for many reasons chocolate should be studiously avoided. Try carob instead, from your health store — a substitute for chocolate.

Researchers at Cornell University in Ithaca, New York, have invented a new method of measuring blood pressure. The technique — recording sound waves in your vascular system — is far superior and more reliable than the traditional arm cuff. With the recorded sound waves, doctors get a visual image that can be analyzed and "read" at a glance.

Stroke

The medical term for stroke is "cerebrovascular accident." A stroke is assuredly not an accident. It is the direct result of a slow buildup of wrong foods coupled with the tense lifestyle most of us live. These impair the circulation of blood, harden arteries and clog the system with deadly waste deposits and toxins. The brain requires a considerable amount of oxygen-fresh blood. A stroke occurs when the circulation of that oxygen to the brain is cut off or interrupted. When the brain does not receive a necessary supply of oxygen through the bloodstream, nerve cells begin to die, causing hemorrhaging or rupture of a blood vessel in the brain.

A stroke may also be caused by *thrombosis* — a blood clot floating in the bloodstream which enters the brain. Because arteries and blood vessels in the brain may be obstructed or thickened, the blood clot may plug an important artery, resulting in a stroke. Or an *embolism* may occur which is the obstruction of a blood vessel by a foreign particle. An *aneurysm* may occur, which is the sudden expansion and breaking of a weak spot in the cerebral (brain) blood vessel. Any of these conditions could have been triggered by too much refined salt, sugar and flour over a period of years, or too little potassium in the diet.

Up to 300,000 crippling, often fatal, strokes could be prevented each year in the U.S. if people recognized the body's early warning signals and sought treatment. "Recent surveys have found that somewhere between 40 and 70% of all people who suffered strokes had some early warning symptoms," revealed Dr. Clark H. Millikan, professor of neurology at the University of Utah School of Medicine, who emphasized: "I think 90% who recognize the symptoms are going to prevent stroke by getting appropriate treatment."

Strokes could be prevented with drugs in most cases, Dr. Millikan said, if people took action based on early warning signs and obtained the proper treatment for high blood pressure. "Many major strokes are preceded by little strokes, warning signals, experienced days, weeks, or months before the more severe event," said American Heart Association (AHA) spokesman Bob Killian. He listed these early-warning signs that often signal an impending, major stroke:

- Sudden, temporary weakness or numbness of the face, arm or leg;
- Temporary dimness or loss of vision, particularly

in one eye;

- Temporary speech difficulty or loss of speech, or trouble understanding speech;
- An episode of double vision;
- Unexplained headaches, or a change in the pattern of your headaches;
- A change in personality or mental ability;
- Warning episodes called Transient Ischemic Attacks, or TIAs, which occur when blood flow to the brain is temporarily interrupted, are almost always due to hardening of the arteries. Symptoms include dizziness, inability to find the right words when talking, blurry vision, slurring of speech, drowsiness, loss of memory, numbness of various parts of the body and paralysis. Most TIAs last two to 15 minutes and nearly all show evidence of clearing up in 12 hours with complete recovery in 24 hours. Of all TIAs, about 1/3 never recur, another 1/3 recur but have no more serious outcome, and the remaining 1/3 are followed sooner or later by a stroke.

The AHA recommends that if you experience one or more of these warning signs, you should immediately see your doctor, who will put you on some sort of drug. Ask your doctor about *Ticlopidine*. Research proves it to be highly effective in preventing strokes. But Dr. Som would advise you to also change to a vegetarian diet and remain on it the rest of your life. Daily in the beginning, and later twice a week, take a warm tub bath with 1/2 teaspoon of cayenne pepper and 1/2 teaspoon of mustard in the bath water. During this twenty minute tub soak, take a cayenne capsule with a cup of warm water, but not on an empty stomach if your stomach is sensitive. It will help you perspire. Take lecithin daily the rest of your life. Order Hanna Kroeger's Circu-Flow and stay on it the rest of your life. You may never need to take the drug.

Ultrasonic Heart Scan and Strokes — There is a simple and inexpensive test that can be given in a physician's office to determine whether or not you are a candidate for a stroke. It is a quick *ultrasonic heart scan*. It does not require injections, catheters or dyes. The ultrasonic scan bounces sound waves off the heart. When the waves react upon the ultrasonic probe, a picture of the heart muscle appears on a screen. If the muscle is thick, you are a candidate. If it is normal, you are not. It's as simple as that. The scan requires only about half an hour. It should cost around $250.00.

If you are a candidate, it may be advisable to change your diet and take certain medications to reduce the risk of stroke. Electrocardiograms are often taken, too, but this method isn't always accurate. The sound wave test is considered more accurate.

Varicose Veins — Varicose veins are a common complaint. What are they and how do they come about? Our first thought perceives that it may be a matter of circulation. The first indication of varicose vein is a dull aching pain. The vein becomes larger, knotted and distended. In extreme cases a rupture of the wall sometimes follows. This is infrequent, but always possible. It is often extremely painful.

The following brief description of the venous system is a summary of the subject, omitting the technical and scientific terms so that the description may be readily understood. Familiarizing ourselves with blood circulation, we realize our heart is constantly pumping fresh oxygenated blood through millions of arteries and capillaries. The blood, leaving the heart, travels all the way to the feet, gathering impurities as it goes. The heart must then pump blood, thick with impurities, back to the heart to be purified again, pulling the blood upward through the veins against the pull of gravity.

The veins are the vessels which serve to return the blood from the capillaries of the different parts of the body to the heart. They are found in nearly every tissue of the body. They are larger and more numerous than arteries, hence the entire capacity of the venous system is much greater than the arterial. Veins have thinner walls than arteries and are not so well supplied with muscular fiber. Hence they are more liable to distension at any point where stagnation is liable to occur.

Two different kinds of veins run through our bodies and varicose veins occur most often in the legs. One large vein runs down the center of the leg, deep inside. Smaller veins run on the outside of the leg, not far beneath the surface. It's these outside veins that usually become varicose, which means twisted. The veins are not only twisted, they are elongated, knotty, hardened and diseased.

All of the larger veins are provided with valves which serve to prevent the reflux of the blood. They are attached by their convex edges to the walls of the veins. Their concave margins are free and directed in the course of the venous current. They lie in close opposition with the wall of the vein as long as the current of blood takes its natural course. If, however, any stagnation or regurgitation occurs, the valves at that point become distorted, their opposed edges are brought into contact, the current is intercepted, and a distension of the wall of the vein ensues.

This distension we know as that very painful affliction, a varicose vein. When the little valves inside the veins which open and close to allow the blood to pass on its journey to the heart fail to function, varicose veins result. The hardened and knotted areas result from patches of clotted blood and chalky deposits on the vein wall, inflaming the lining of the vein.

You create some of your own problems, usually by standing or sitting in the same position for long periods of time. When you are forced to stand, you should walk around and exercise the circulation. Standing still in the same position for long periods causes blood to stagnate and valves to cease to function. Movement and exercise aids in keeping the blood moving along its upward journey and helps the valves to close properly. Movement and exercise also intake good oxygen which, entering the bloodstream, helps to purify it. There are so many occasions for standing in our modern life — in line at the market, waiting for a bus, on a crowded bus. Dentists, barbers, beauty operators, workers "at the bench," and salespersons find themselves standing for long periods. If this is true in your case, then find ways to move around and to sit often.

There are also occasions when we must sit for long periods — on the bus, a plane trip, or even at our desks. If you would prevent varicose veins, you must rise occasionally, walk around or do something to create circulation. The quiescent upright position of the desk worker produces stagnation of the blood in the legs, hence pressure and a steady strain upon the walls of the venous system at that point. Result, a permanent distension or "varicose veins." In youth, if a change of occupation is made, this affliction may disappear. But if the trouble occurs in or after middle age, a cure by any lotion or other medicinal remedy is difficult. Look first to nutrition and lack of exercise.

As the primal cause of the trouble is stagnation of the blood, acceleration of the circulation would relieve that congestion, and an excellent method is by friction, according to Sanford Bennett. The most effective method for accomplishing this is with the dry palms of the hands, and the most convenient time and place is in bed in the early morning, before you arise. The conditions are then favorable as the system is relaxed and will readily respond to intelligently directed efforts towards its rejuvenation and improvement. The trouble will most probably appear on the inside of the leg below the knee, running along the path of the leg. But it may extend several inches above the knee and along the inside of the thigh. With increase in age, the congestion or distension of the superficial veins will extend lower down, immediately above and around the ankle. This may become discolored and assume a deep bluish hue, because of the stagnant blood.

Relief is obtained by friction with the palm daily and persistently. The friction will relieve the congestion, strengthen the minute muscles that support the venous walls and, if persisted in systematically and methodically, will finally restore the distorted venous valves to their proper position, and the trouble will disappear. It is a simple, easy, and effective remedy for a very annoying affliction.

The most convenient position is lying on your side. Commence with 20 strokes of the hand up and down, following the course of the vein, increasing to 100 strokes as the skin becomes hardened and accustomed to the friction. If persisted in, a cure is ultimately sure in any ordinary case. So says Sanford Bennett. May I add that applying Tea Tree Oil or cold pressed castor oil along with all that friction would probably aid considerably in the healing of these distorted veins.

Many people find that massaging with Fanie's Oak Bark Cleanser is very beneficial because of its natural DMSO and other excellent natural ingredients. See the last chapter for where to order.

Adding the research of Dr. Som's to that of Sanford Bennett, he said your diet must include an adequate supply of vitamin C. A deficiency in vitamin C seems to be a major cause of varicose veins. Vitamin P — also known as flavonoids, rutin and hesperidin — is also essential. Vitamin E is certainly required for the health of the blood vessels. Swollen veins have been known to totally disappear with the intake of massive doses of vitamin E.

If your job requires standing or sitting all day, do try to find time during the day to lie down with your feet higher than your head — on a slant board, if possible. Or put blocks under the foot of your bed to raise your feet higher than your head all through the night.

Congestion of the liver is frequently a cause of varicose veins. Vitamin B complex is essential for this problem. Brewer's yeast tablets, containing all the vitamin B complex, are excellent to detoxify the liver. *Collinsonia root* is a good herbal remedy. And *cayenne herb capsules* will perform wonders in circulation. Certainly a change in diet is essential. Toss out your white sugar, salt and flour — and processed foods. This is a beginning. (See *The Book of Beginning Again* for further guidelines.)

Dr. Som always advised his varicose patients to walk or run backward in water — in a swimming pool, in a homemade backyard water tank or Jacuzzi, or even your bathtub. The water preferably should not rise over the height of the thighs, but can reach waist high. The important thing is for there to be water pressure against the calves. In this hydrotherapy massage, the legs should be lifted high as you walk backward. Lie on a slant board afterward to elevate your feet above the level of your head. This helps release pressure of the blood in the veins. Dr. Som also taught leg exercises and guidelines:

1) while standing pigeon-toed raise up and down on your toes;

2) tense the leg muscles tightly with your feet together, forcing the calves against each other;

3) lie on your back and stretch the toes toward your head, thereby stretching the tendons of Achilles in the lower leg;

4) temporary relief may be obtained by the use of elastic stockings, but continuing your occupation will cause a reoccurrence of the problem;

5) the secretary must find occasions to rise and walk around and the beauty operator must find occasions to sit;

6) tight clothing, tight garters, and tight girdles restrict the flow of blood. For the one prone to varicose veins, they should be avoided;

7) do not sleep with one leg atop the other. Circulation is impeded in every part of the body;

8) try applying undiluted apple cider vinegar every morning and evening. It's an old European folk medicine used to alleviate varicose veins.

These suggestions are certainly better than resorting to surgery which strips away the swollen veins. The surgeon ties off the veins at each end of the leg so that blood can no longer enter them. Sometimes the surgery is successful, but often it is not. It is not natural for veins to be tied off. It's against nature. Such a procedure can result in additional circulatory problems. It only adds stress to the large vein deep inside the leg. It is far better to attempt a cure the natural way.

If natural approaches fail, in order to avoid surgery, ask your doctor about a new painless technique which often cures. It involves injection with a chemical solution called *sodium tetradecyl sulphate*, which causes the breaks in the walls of the veins to stick together, close and disappear. It can be done in a doctor's office, enabling one to avoid a long expensive hospital stay. But seek the injection or surgery as a very last resort.

Aching Legs — can be relieved by walking exercise. Elevate the legs for half an hour every day which can be done by watching TV lying on a couch with a wedge pillow under your legs. Buy a hand-held vibrator and massage your leg muscles to stimulate circulation, or massage with your hands. Take a warm tub soak if possible. Wear support hose or socks. Make sure your shoes are low heeled and comfortable, with adequate built-in arch supports. Discard white salt which retains fluid, causing swelling in the legs. If your work requires standing, make sure a hard surface is covered by a cushioned or rubber mat.

Crossed Legs — Never cross your legs at the knees. Dr. Som said this is one of the greatest sins against blood circulation. It causes varicose veins. And it throws the lower spine out of alignment, causing backache. Prop up your feet when possible. Lie on a slant board often.

Dangers of a Long Air Flight — A report has just been published in the prestigious international medical journal *The Lancet* with a warning that flying in a plane longer than three hours can kill you. Sitting in a cramped airplane seat can create blood clots in your legs that, breaking off, could lodge in your heart or lungs. You must walk around the cabin once an hour. You must do simple exercises such as flexing your legs, stretching them, lifting them, holding and then dropping them. Stand and raise up on your toes several times. Drink a lot of water. Do not drink alcohol. It dehydrates you and thickens the blood. If you smoke, space out your pattern. Smoking could increase the formation of blood clots.

Electric Heating Blankets — Toss them away! When you warm the body artificially night after night you are causing the body's own thermo-genetic apparatus to turn off, blocking your flow of circulation. Dr. Som said the body's own heating mechanism would cease to function if you constantly heat the body artificially. Not only that but the artificial heat causes inflammation throughout the muscles, increasing difficulties of arthritis, inflammation, infection, low back aches and weakened muscles.

Why not try other methods. If you sleep with cold feet, why not a pair of socks? Why not cotton flannel pajamas and flannel sheets next to the body, covered with a thermal blanket, with another blanket atop that, which will help the body create its own heat and hold it inside the covers. Or buy a down-filled cotton comforter.

If you *must* have a heated bed, turn the electric blanket on a few moments before retiring, just to warm the bed. When you retire, turn it off. Your own body heat will then take over and, with the help of the thermal blanket, you should stay warm. Also, a cayenne herbal capsule at bedtime will start the blood circulating, not only for warmth but for good health. A cup of warm whole raw milk at bedtime, with its natural tryptophane, should assure a good nights sleep. If you can't buy raw milk, forget it. Homogenized could lead to a heart attack.

Phlebitis — Dr. Som suggested taking 1,000 milligrams of vitamin C every hour for two days when fighting colds, flu, or phlebitis. Then reduce to 2000 mgs. a day. Reduce further for daily use. Don't stay on such a megadose indefinitely. Taking megadoses of vitamin C for an extended period and then stopping suddenly can be hazardous. The body, recognizing an overdose, begins releasing enzymes that destroy the excessive vitamin. If you suddenly cease the massive doses, the enzymes continue to flow for several months, attacking the normal intake of vitamin C, causing a deficiency. During this time of vitamin C deficiency, you are subject to flu, colds and other infections. So taper off the massive doses gradually to resume the daily intake of around 70 mgs. The enzymes will then adjust to the normal intake.

Also take a daily vitamin E capsule, 400 units. Continue vitamin C and E tablets the rest of your life to keep the veins toned. Also take bioflavonoid and rutin tablets for strengthening the veins. Change to a vegetarian diet. During a flare-up of inflammation, fast on fruit and vegetable juices only, with an occasional bowl of fresh vegetable broth. Apply alternating hot and cold packs over the inflammation. Walk in water, even if it's only in your bathtub, as cold as tolerable.

Medical Advances

Now let's see what wonders the medical establishment is offering to aid in the struggle to "clear the arteries." The National Science Foundation reports that microscopic scraping machines called micromoters have been developed at the University of California at Berkeley. No wider than a human hair, they will travel up and down your arteries clearing away fatty deposits that lead to heart attacks and strokes.

Doctors at Montifiore Hospital in New York report that an amazing new "smart laser" can remove the hardened debris in the arteries without damaging healthy tissue. This enables doctors to save arms and legs that otherwise might have to be amputated. The laser beams its destructive ray only when it meets an obstruction in the artery, vaporizing fat deposits.

al Milano — In a tiny mountain hamlet in northern Italy, an amazing protein has been found that destroys cholesterol deposits in veins and arteries. The inhabitants of this Italian village suffer very little heart problem and live well into their hundreds. Researchers expect to have an artificial version of the protein available soon but the new protein itself may not be available until the mid-1990s. The protein is called *al Milano*. The drug acts as a scavenger to destroy cholesterol in the blood vessels.

Aneurysm — When a blood vessel balloons inside the brain, it's called an aneurysm. An aneurysm can cause a spasm. A drug called *Nimotop* can eliminate the spasm. Nimotop also reduces nerve damage created by the aneurysm.

Blood Clots — There is now a drug called *Streptokinase* and another called *tPA* which are given to dissolve blood clots. Either of these is given during an acute heart attack, or when one threatens. The medication dissolves blood clots and restores the flow of blood through the arteries. A new drug called *Eminase* has been successful in dissolving blood clots. And if injected within a few hours of an attack, it improves the possibility of survival.

Capoten — is the name of a new drug accomplishing astonishing results in patients with congestive heart failure. Do ask your doctor about it.

Cardene — This drug can be used to treat a patient in the initial stage of a heart attack. It lowers blood pressure and stabilizes an irregular heartbeat.

Cemfibrozil — From Finland comes a report of excellent results from the use of a drug called *Cemfibrozil*, which reduced the level of harmful cholesterol and triglycerides while simultaneously raising the amount of good cholesterol.

Leech Saliva — Who'd ever think the lowly leech would enter the medical scene again! The ancients who used leeches for practically every ailment knew a secret we're just now discovering — the saliva of leeches contains a chemical substance that thins the blood and dissolves blood clots. The biologists call it *herudin*. It's injected into the bloodstream of patients threatened by fatal blood clots. It sweeps rapidly through the body dissolving the clots that form during a stroke or heart attack and promises to save many lives.

MK-801 — On the horizon is a new drug to battle the damage done by heart attacks and strokes. The drug wards off crippling brain damage. When a stroke or heart attack strikes, the flow of blood to the brain is usually blocked, causing brain cells to die because they lack oxygen. But the new drug, *MK-801*, appears to be able to revive the cells, even if given 24 hours after the attack. Tests with animals have proven almost one hundred percent effective in protecting and rejuvenating affected brain cells.

The Myoglobin Test — is a simple new blood test replacing an expensive and risky surgical technique now being used to determine if special clot-dissolving drugs are actually dissolving the clots. This new myoglobin test is replacing coronary arteriography, which involves snaking a catheter with a scope and lens through blood vessels to discover if the clots have dissolved.

Niacin (vitamin B3) — reduces high cholesterol in the blood and raises the level of needed cholesterol. It impedes hardening of the arteries. But don't take it before checking with your doctor. Diabetics, ulcer patients and several other types could be harmed.

The Infamous Pacemaker — Don't be easily persuaded to have a pacemaker "installed." A new study reveals that one in five is unnecessary. A pacemaker is often prescribed by doctors who aren't even heart specialists. A change in diet may prove far more effective. Not only that, about 30,000 patients need to have their pacemakers replaced every year because of wear and tear or defects in the device. Manufacturers of these defective devices can't be forced to replace their product even if they're still under warranty. So if a pacemaker is suggested, seek a second opinion before submitting. Consider chelation instead.

Heart Transplants — sometimes dubbed a great medical progress — are very much in the news these years. But why not try healing the heart you have, instead of relying on a transplant of another person's heart? Because if you continue the lifestyle that caused your own heart to collapse then your new heart surely will, too, sooner or later. So why not visit a chiropractor or an osteopath to have the nerves unpinched, discard your white sugar, flour, salt and all processed foods and start doing yoga and deep breathing exercise. Start to regenerate your own body.

You can't expect your doctor to know much about it. He is only trained in drug therapy — that is, unless you are fortunate enough to find a new breed of doctor, a holistic physician. Then — lucky you — he may be able to guide you into a whole new way of life. If physicians would only learn how to guide people toward natural therapy, perhaps heart disease would soon be virtually unknown.

Vasatec — is also effective in lowering high blood pressure. It will also reduce fluid buildup around the heart.

Vision Heart Analyzer — There is a new test available now in many doctor's offices which can help predict whether you are a candidate for a heart attack within the next six years. The test is called the *Vision Blood Analyzer.* The procedure is to draw a small sample of your blood and run it through the blood analyzer computer which does a complete analysis of your blood, including the levels of fats, cholesterol and glucose. Then the doctor will record your blood pressure in the computer, whether or not you smoke and whether or not you have diabetes. He will enter your age and sex. Shortly thereafter, the computer should print out a reading which will advise whether or not you face a life threatening heart attack, or whether or not changes should be made in your diet and lifestyle.

The test is available in the offices of many doctors, but if your doctor is not familiar with the procedure, have him contact for further information: Customer Service, Abbott Laboratories, Abbott Park, Illinois 60064.

What Happened to EG-626? — I have an old yellowed newspaper clipping describing the efforts of Dr. Takio Shimamoto, Professor Emeritus at Tokyo Medical and Dental University and Director of the Japan Arteriosclerosis Research Institute. The clipping says he has released a report on twenty years of medical research attempting to find a drug that will prevent heart attacks and strokes. He says that he has at last developed such a drug. He calls it a breakthrough. United States government scientists at the National Institute of Health have shown considerable interest in his work. Dr. Shimamoto states:

"This is the medical breakthrough for heart attacks and

strokes that I've been working on for twenty years. The new drug — called EG-626 (EG for short) — cleanses the blood vessels of thromboxane A2, a substance manufactured naturally by the body which causes arteries to clog up.

"It neutralizes the deadly thromboxane A2 and rejuvenates arteries that have hardened. The effect of EG is almost immediate and it has shown no side effects in our experiments. When we administer EG to those who have had heart attacks or strokes or appear on the verge of doing so, they cease to register their symptoms. EG counteracts the effects of thromboxane in only minutes. Therefore, there are no heart attacks or strokes and the continued cleansing prevents them in the future. More than five hundred Japanese who are prone to heart attacks or strokes are undergoing tests at this moment. I feel there is an extremely promising chance the drug will be on the Japanese market soon."

Dr. Shimamoto goes on to explain that out of five hundred people taking the tasteless, colorless drug in pill form daily, none have suffered a heart attack or stroke except those who stopped taking the EG. One man, he said, took EG for a year, stopped taking it and had a heart attack. He went back on the drug and is now working harder than ever. A 72-year-old business man from southwestern Japan suffered from chest pains and dizziness and had to give up golf because of hardening of the arteries. After only one month on EG the chest pains disappeared and he was able to play golf again.

Other doctors in Japan also involved in the study of EG are Dr. Fujio Numano, Associate Professor of Medicine at Tokyo Medical and Dental University. He states, "I have been involved in the study of EG and I feel this is one of the biggest breakthroughs in heart and stroke medicine in two decades." Dr. T. K. Zemplenyi, Professor of Medicine at the University of Southern California School of Medicine in Los Angeles, a cardiologist doing research into arteriosclerosis stated, "Dr. Shimamoto is one of the great men in the study of arteriosclerosis internationally accepted."

Dr. Donald Fry, Chief of the Laboratory of Experimental Arteriosclerosis at the National Heart, Lung and Blood Institute in Bethesda, Maryland, has sponsored two seminars in order to hear more of Dr. Shimamoto's work. He stated, "If his results can be duplicated in the United States, I'm sure it could have a tremendous life-saving impact in the areas of heart attack and stroke which annually claim the lives of at least a million Americans."

Well, to repeat, that newspaper clipping is now yellowed with age. It isn't dated, but it must be several years old. I wonder whatever happened to EG-626. Americans continue to have serious heart attacks and strokes. They submit daily by the thousands to surgery to unplug the arteries or have bypasses or have a new heart installed. If EG-626 was so wonderful, why didn't we start using it here? Is it now being successfully used in Japan? If so, what happened? Did our FDA turn it down? If so, why? Why hasn't our own research included it? If it is all the tests indicate, why do Americans keep dying by the millions with our number one killer? Why should we submit to such agonizing therapy if there is a better method? Whatever happened to EG-626? If anyone knows, please notify me. I'd like to know — and I'm sure my readers would, too.

Chapter Eleven

Tumors and Cancer

If diet obviously is involved in such diseases as heart problems and diabetes, surely it must be obvious that the diet is also involved in cancer diseases. Our diet and our daily habits — whether or not we smoke or overindulge in alcohol — and the location of our homesite which involves smog pollutants, are all involved in cancer. The role of diet is particularly important in the prevention and healing of cancer. Tobacco is too obvious a role to require a further warning.

Anal Cancer — A large majority of patients with anal cancer are now able to avoid surgery and the accompanying colostomy bag thanks to the use of two new cancer fighting drugs, *5-FU* and *Mitomycin-C*, combined with radiation therapy. This new approach is not only saving lives, but improving the quality of the lives being saved as well, according to Dr. Ben Sischy, clinical professor of oncology at the University of Rochester, and Dr. Julian Ambrus, director of cancer research at Roswell Park Memorial Institute.

Bone Cancer — Doctors in China surgically remove diseased bone, treat it and return it to the body, resulting, eventually, in a total cure.

Brain Tumor — Famous healer Hanna Kroeger writes that she applied a poultice of mashed raw tomatoes to her child's head when a brain tumor was suspected. She changed the mass of mashed raw tomatoes every six hours. She continued this procedure for seven days. After the third day the child's severe headaches left and on the seventh day normalcy returned. She states that after the fourth application a horrible odor penetrated the room and after completing the treatment she discarded all the bed clothing because the odor had penetrated everything; but the suspected brain tumor had disappeared.

Hanna now says a tofu poultice is even more effective than the tomatoes. Just mashed tofu, which can be purchased at any health store. Do write Hanna directly for further details. Address in last chapter.

Breast Tumors — Quick removal of breast tumors is being researched at Thomas Jefferson University in Philadelphia. The new method involves portable sonar devices that can pinpoint tumors with extreme accuracy. Once the sonar unit locates the site of the tumor, the sonar device then removes the growth without damaging surrounding tissues, as the surgeon often does when he must probe to locate the tumor.

Many patients are also opting for the removal of just the breast lump plus radiation treatment. This leaves the breast itself intact, and the treatment is equally as effective as radical mastectomy — the removal of the entire breast. It is no longer necessary to have the radical mastectomy once performed on all women. The doctor is required to advise you of all your options and alternative procedures.

It's good that doctors can no longer automatically perform a total mastectomy when a tiny cancerous lump appears. They are required by law now to enlighten the patient about radiotherapy in which only the cancerous tissue is removed. Then the patient is free to choose the methodology *she* prefers.

There is now a relatively inexpensive device on the market which can be a tremendous step forward in helping women detect lumps in their breasts while they are still extremely tiny. It is called a *Sensor Pad* and it works like a "finger stethoscope." The silicone-lubricated latex pad is placed over the breast to amplify the sense of touch, thus enabling the woman to detect lumps no bigger than a human hair. The Sensor Pad was developed by the Inventive Products Co. in Decatur, Illinois and sells for about $15.

Alcohol has been linked to breast cancer. Even moderate drinkers increase the risk of breast cancer. Knowing the risk involved should make it easy to become a teetotaler. Caffeine also triggers lumps in the breast, although some are benign. If you have benign lumps, better give up all caffeine. It can turn the benign tumors into cancerous growths.

There is a product called *PM-7* which heals fibrocystic breast disease and prostate problems, both of which are caused by a buildup of cholesterol in the breasts and in the prostate. It binds with sterols, thus is effective in removing accumulated cholesterol from the system, whether in the arteries or in the breast tissues. The removal of cholesterol also prevents heart attacks and strokes. Fibrocystic breast disease is no more than cysts formed on the breasts as a result of too much cholesterol. The breast is a major manufacturing site of cholesterol in women. These cysts are usually benign but frequently they undergo a chemical change, combining with oxygen to form cholesterol oxide, just as iron combines with oxygen to form rust. Cholesterol oxide is a carcinogen, that is, it causes breast cancer. Thus anyone with cysts on the breast or enlargement of the prostate would do well to take the product PM-7 to reduce the buildup of cholesterol throughout the body. It is obtainable by writing Health Information Service. (Address elsewhere).

A book called *Cholesterols: Causing Cancers and A Whole Lot More* can be obtained through Health Information Service. It will answer fully all questions concerning the removal of cholesterols without undergoing surgery.

The Surgeon General's new Report on Nutrition and Health emphasizes a reduction of fat in the diet. Apparently fat increases the risk of breast cancer. It is certain that fatty acids directly activate tumor-cell growth.

Calcium Blocker — At the Arizona Cancer Center in Tucson, tests are proving a calcium-blocking drug called *Verapamil* helps to prevent cancer cells from becoming resistant to standard chemotherapy.

Cancer Detecting Blood Test — Researchers at Beth Israel Hospital in Boston have discovered a simple new blood test which can spot cancer in its earliest stages. The blood is run through a *magnetic resonance imaging* machine called an MRI. The MRI detects cancer at such an early stage the patients are not aware of any problems, nor would the doctors have been able to detect the cancer through the conventional methods of testing. Such a device could make the regular annual checkup include a simple cancer detecting blood test.

Cervical Cancer — There is new hope for women with cervical cancer. Researchers at Birmingham University in England report that a mixture of two drugs, *Bleomycin* and *Cisplatin*, has cured or remarkably improved cervical cancer in thousands of women. Those who weren't completely cured were able to be cured with radiation therapy after taking the mixture.

Fibroid Tumors — A new procedure called *hysteroscopic surgery* is eliminating the need for major surgery. Fibroid tumors, which are growths on the muscle of the uterus, cause pain, bleeding, and infertility. The usual procedure has been a hysterectomy. The new procedure dilates the cervix and instruments fed through the hysteroscope removes the tumors. The whole technique requires only about an hour and the patient often returns to work the following day. This is extremely important news for women and is long overdue.

Head and Neck Cancer — is now being treated nonsurgically. The new treatment alternates between a week of radiation and chemotherapy with a week of no treatments. The week of rest gives the normal cells a chance to recover. Why not also take Laetrile tablets, and Tribalene herb capsules made by Jason Winters which he claims healed him of mouth and neck cancer?

Interferon — is a cellular protein which is produced when a viral infection occurs in a cell. Its job is to prevent the reproduction of the virus. A substance similar to the natural interferon produced by your body is now being used to fight cancer.

Lung Cancer — High doses of vitamin B have been found to reduce precancerous cells in the lungs. B vitamins taken in tincture form under the tongue are even more effective. They may be ordered from Fanie International. See the last chapter for name and address of distributors.

Magic Bullets — Scientists at the Molecular Biology Laboratory report that they are successfully treating cancer patients by targeting *monoclonal antibodies*, known as "magic bullets" against cancer cells. The antibodies help the immune system recognize and destroy cancer cells.

Oral Cancer — Researchers at Harvard University are using an extract of common algae to heal cancer of the mouth. The extract seems to stimulate the immune system into high gear, enabling the body to fight the tumor by itself.

Ovarian Cancer — A new ultrasonic method now being used by obstetricians/gynecologists offers promise of more positive and earlier detection of ovarian cancer. An ultrasonic probe is inserted in the vagina. It emits high-frequency sound waves which project a picture of the ovaries on a TV like screen. If the ovaries are enlarged it indicates they may be cancerous. It's a simple, painless, five-minute probe and may save thousands of women from death, states Dr. Hellen Rodriquez and Dr. Lawrence Platt, who are conducting the study at the University of Southern California. Any obstetrician/gynecologist can conduct the test, which could be done along with a woman's yearly Pap test. All women past menopause are potential candidates.

Prostate Cancer — The prostate is a small donut-shaped gland found only in men. It's located just below the bladder near the rectum. Its purpose is to produce a zinc-rich substance which becomes a part of the semen. It can occasionally cause trouble because its location exposes it to bacterial infection and inflammation. It naturally enlarges with age. It can become cancerous as men age. It should be carefully checked during every physical exam, which should occur yearly in men over 40.

Ultrasound is now being used to examine and to treat prostate cancer. The imaging is obtained by inserting a sound-emitting probe into the rectum. The image is then recorded on a laser disk. Such a method enables the doctor to treat the problem with the correct placement of cancer-destructive radioactive seeds. It reduces the risk of nerve damage and impaired sexual activities.

Symptoms to watch for, which indicate possible problems, are: blood in the urine; frequent or urgent urination; a weak stream of urination; loss of bladder control resulting in incontinence; pain or burning during urination; pain in lower back, pelvis or upper thighs; inability to pass urine. If cancer is suspect during the annual rectal examination, the doctor uses a needle to remove a minuscule sample of prostate tissue for testing. It's almost painless. If the tissue test proves positive, the usual procedure is removal of the testicles to reduce the level of male hormone testosterone, or to treat with drugs.

If the cancer is detected before it spreads it can be cured through surgery or radiation therapy. If not, there is no known cure. Cause of prostate cancer seems difficult to pinpoint, but diet surely could be involved, especially too much fat. Also contact Michael Tierra or Hanna Kroeger for possible herbal remedies. Don't accept the verdict of "no known cure."

Sandostatin — is a drug now being used to fight the diarrhea that can be caused by intestinal cancer.

Skin Cancer — Signals to watch for are: moles that change shape, color or texture; moles that become painful, itchy or which bleed. A mole that has an irregular or ragged border. A mole that divides in color, one half not matching the other. A mottled colored mole. A mole wider than 1/4 inch.

Patients with metastatic melanoma, a deadly form of skin cancer, may soon be dramatically healed. A new type of treatment involves draining a patient's blood, heating it, mixing it with the anti-cancer drug *Melphalem* and returning it to the body. The results have been so dramatic the doctors involved in the treatment intimate it may even lead to a vaccine for cancer.

It is reported that Retin-A, the now renowned anti-wrinkle face cream, protects against skin cancer. It banishes actinic keratoses, precancerous growths, and even blocks the development of melanoma, the deadly form of skin cancer mentioned above. So claim several manufacturers.

Garlic and Skin Cancer — Is there a natural alternative to surgery and other conventional methods of removal? Well, an article in the news recently told how Kirby Allan of Mesa, Arizona, cured skin cancer using garlic. The cancer appeared on the tip of his nose and remained for years. His wife urged him to have the traditional cancer surgery but he refused. Instead he mashed some garlic, spread it on a Band-Aid and applied it to the sore. He changed the dressing four times in ten days. After the first two days the garlic raised the sore, then drew pus. A day later, it started to drain. Then the skin started flaking. He kept it covered another week. By then the sore had healed over.

He next applied the garlic to a suspicious mole on his hip. It simply fell off. Doctors aware of his self-healing readily admit to the incredible potent chemical in garlic which has been used to stop colon cancer. If you have a skin cancer problem, why not discuss it with your doctor and experiment?

Sunspots — There's a new "wrinkle" to help one avoid skin cancer, which is usually caused by overexposure to the sun. It's a device called Sunspots — tiny adhesive bandages that, stuck on the skin, turn blue when the skin has had enough harmful ultraviolet light.

Sneakers and Cancer — A new research reveals that the insoles used in sport shoes of all kinds contain two chemicals — called MBT and DBTD — that cause cancer. The chemicals are used by rubber manufacturers to harden their products. When the feet sweat, these chemicals are absorbed into the bloodstream. MBT is also used in rubber linings of our refrigerators, in bottle caps, in jars and food containers and in infant tennis shoes. The FDA has only recently ordered it removed from pacifiers and baby bottle nipples.

Dr. Jerry McLaughlin of Purdue University, a research scientist, and Dr. Jere Guin of the University of Arkansas Medical School, warn that if tennis shoes cause your feet to itch, swell, blister or ache — or even if they don't — you'd better stop wearing sneakers. Because it only takes one molecule of a carcinogen to trigger cancer.

Stomach Tumors — Dr. Som was renowned for his stomach cures, especially tumors. He was not a great one to put people on a strict water fast, except for curing stomach tumors. That's when he said the stomach must not be given work to do, so he asked the patient to stop eating. He gave them half a tablespoon of pure fresh lemon juice and a little water twice a day. At other times he insisted on drinking only distilled water. He gave the patient nourishment through the rectum and through oil rubs, especially sesame or olive oil. He also insisted on exercising in sunshine and fresh air. He prepared a liquid bowel food thusly:

He filled a jar half full of oatmeal. Sometimes it was pure steel-cut grain oatmeal, sometimes it was rolled oats.

He filled the remainder of the jar to the top so that he had half oatmeal and half water. He allowed it to stand overnight and the next morning he strained out a cupful of the liquid. He heated it to body temperature and injected it through the rectum by a regular rectal syringe. The intestines and bowels went to work absorbing the nutrition in this liquid food while the stomach stayed quiet. He injected this liquid food twice a day.

He oiled and massaged the complete body morning and evening. After covering the entire body with either sesame or olive oil he insisted the patient expose the body to fresh air, preferably air with early morning sunshine. He said the bloodstream absorbed nutrition from the oil through the skin. During the fresh air bath the patient was told to take slow, deep breaths along with simple exercises. The fresh air bath was followed by a warm shower and finished off with a few seconds of cold, unless the cold was too shocking.

If running bowels became a problem, making the rectum a bit raw, he applied olive oil or castor oil to the tender parts. He said the poisons emitting from the body might tend to create running bowels, because the bowels were evacuating considerable toxins and phlegm.

This program continued for about three weeks, then he gave a little raw food, a small salad. If the food caused pain in the stomach, he resumed the liquid diet until the tumor was completely healed. If after three weeks there was no pain, he continued to give small quantities of salad until the patient slowly returned to a normal diet. Even then he continued the fast on alternate days — one day on foods, the next day on liquids, for a week or two. Or two days on liquids and one on solids.

If patients couldn't endure the water fast he had them simply eat live, raw foods (salads) in moderation for a long period. This prevented the necessity for a fast at all. It took longer to heal but the patients certainly got well on it. So said Dr. Som.

Testicle Cancer — is now being treated with an effective drug called *Ifex*. But since it often results in unpleasant side effects, *Mesnex* is used to reduce and counteract those side effects. A new surgical operation keeps the nerves intact, which means fatherhood is still possible — as opposed to the old conventional type of testicle surgery. Good news for many patients!

For more information concerning cancer of any kind call the toll-free "hot line" number in the last chapter. And to get a free copy of a useful booklet *50 Fast Facts To Reduce Your Risk of Cancer*, send a self-addressed business-size envelope with 65 cents in postage to: M.D. Anderson Cancer Center, Dept. of Cancer Prevention/189, 1515 Holcombe, Houston, Texas 77030.

Cancer and Jason Winters — Now that I have given both conventional and nonconventional approaches to avoiding or healing cancer, I must refer you to the writings of Jason Winters which tell the story of his battle against cancer and the conventional approach, of his rejection of such an approach, and of how he overcame cancer with Laetrile and herbs. I've mentioned it already but it bears repeating. Do purchase his book *Killing Cancer* at your health store or order from Swanson's (address elsewhere). The book describes his incredible experience. And if you are a cancer patient he offers guidelines toward a possible cure.

Winters describes his change to a vegetarian diet and he encourages exercising. He suggests taking pancreatic enzymes just prior to taking Laetrile. The enzymes can also be obtained through VitaChem. It enables the Laetrile (apricot kernels) to work more effectively. His

Tribalene herbal capsules contain three special herbs which, combined, dramatically affect tumors and cancers. He suggests you add asparagus tips to your diet — almost daily. He insists on raw vegetable and fruit salads, whole wheat bread only, twenty raw almonds daily, five pancreatic enzymes before each meal. Drink fresh carrot juice. Take four 500 mg. Laetrile (Amygdalin) tablets daily. He suggests coffee enemas often (see his book for details). Avoid canned goods (except Jolly Green Giant asparagus if unavailable fresh). Avoid white salt and smoking. He suggests potassium tablets daily. He suggests his herbal product Zion to stimulate the thymus.

Winters suggests drinking only distilled water — so did Dr. Som. Both say it acts as a magnet to leech out all the embedded minerals which prevent your cells from performing naturally. You can have a water distiller installed in your home. You may also want to order the free book, *Fifty Fast Facts to Reduce Your Risk of Cancer* just mentioned. One "fast fact" is to take garlic capsules or eat garlic to avoid colon cancer. Also see how garlic was used to heal a serious "nose" cancer. Another: avoid fish oil supplements. But see my suggestion of taking flaxseed oil and flaxseed instead, for many reasons. I take both Laetrile and Tribalene just for preventive measures — one Laetrile tablet daily and one Tribalene daily. I eat five fresh shelled almonds daily. I walk and perform the yogic exercise Salutation to the Sun described in the Degree teachings of Astara's *Book of Life*. I perform the isometric exercises described by Sanford Bennett in my *Book of Beginning Again*. I take an occasional Zion tablet and a pancreatic enzyme (B15). I eat a lot of fresh asparagus. I drink only distilled water. I eat a lot of raw salads and only whole wheat bread. I drink one cup of apple cider vinegar-honey cocktail mentioned earlier to obtain potassium. All these are simply good daily habits which anyone can follow, not only to prevent cancer but simply to maintain good health. None are difficult and easily become a way of life. I am also a vegetarian, which might present difficulties for some people.

Order Laetrile (Amygdalin B 17) from VitaChem (see last chapter) and purchase Tribalene and Zion herb capsules at your health store or order from Swanson's.

Chapter Twelve

Arthritis, Osteoporosis, and Pain

Arthritis

Arthritis and Diet — To your daily intake of vitamin E add a spoonful of flaxseed oil and a capsule of evening primrose oil. The three taken together — vitamin E, flaxseed oil, primrose — reduce inflammation. In tests by scientists at the University of Pennsylvania, primrose oil alone brought vast improvement to rheumatoid arthritics. Evening primrose, like cod liver oil and flaxseed, has a high content of fatty acids which block the effect of certain "bad" chemicals in the body that cause inflammation. Combining it with flaxseed oil and vitamin E could spell the end of arthritis pain. Proven helpful in tests, also, is a combination of vitamin E, selenium and cayenne herb tablets. Be sure the selenium is low dosage if taken daily.

In tests blocking the production of bad chemicals in the body the search of the scientists should be to determine what created "bad" chemicals in the body in the first place. Could it be the diet? It must be because if it was a bad chemical natural to the body then everybody would be subject to the production of said bad chemical — which is not the case. What causes arthritis in some people and not in others? If you're an arthritic, do consider your diet.

Food suggestions: fish cooked in olive oil or canola. Olive or canola oils are each extremely effective in combating inflammation, lubricating swollen joints and destroying pain-causing chemicals, such as prostaglandins. Cook also with onion and garlic. For considerable information concerning arthritis and flaxseed oil, see my book *Forever Young*. It seems redundant to repeat the same information in this book.

Arthritis and Infections — A blood test should reveal the proportion of calcium and phosphorus in the blood. Doctors familiar with arthritis believe the ideal portions are a level of 10 for calcium against a level of 4 for phosphorus. Any alterations of these proportions should be a warning to be watchful for arthritis. Stress can cause an upset in the chemistry. Mechanical conditions can be the cause, such as poor posture, poor sitting habits, bad sleeping habits. If you have experienced a recent infection, do ask your doctor for a blood test to determine the calcium-phosphorus proportion, which can be agitated through an infection. Often eliminating the infection will cause the arthritis to vanish.

If there seems to be a hidden cause of infection, do consider the stumps of tonsils which may have been left from a tonsillectomy. The infected root may be overgrown with scar tissue preventing the proper healing. Thus the infection drains constantly throughout the system. But be very sure of the diagnosis of such tonsil roots.

Many good teeth have been removed without clearly establishing an infected root canal to be the cause of arthritis. Certainly it can be. And if such an infection is suspected, consider having the tooth removed rather than suffering unnecessarily with arthritis. Menopause can often upset the body chemistry and aggravate arthritis. Avoid refined foods and avoid sugars and white flour foods. Sugar is a certain means of upsetting the calcium-phosphorus balance. The apple cider vinegar-honey cocktail has often been suggested to raise the phosphorus level.

Arthritis and Vitamin C — There is every indication that all forms of arthritis result from a lack of vitamin C in the diet. Take it daily to prevent arthritis. If you have a tendency towards any form of arthritis — rheumatic fever, rheumatoid arthritis, primary osteoarthritis, rheumatoid spondylitis, bursitis, etc. — do be sure of your vitamin C intake. If you are already a victim, try taking a thousand milligrams to ten thousands milligrams a day, depending on your individual needs. Discuss it with your doctor.

Vitamin C also prevents infection. Massive doses of vitamin C in injections and orally have been known to bring about complete and rapid cures. Most foods have lost much of their vitamin C by the time they are served at the table. Not only through cooking, but because of our methods of transportation and marketing. Avoid cigarette smoke under all circumstances. It will rob you of vitamin C. Increase your intake of vitamin C if you take aspirin daily, since aspirin leaches vitamin C from your body.

Relieving the Pain of Arthritis

One of the best and effective methods of reducing the pain of rheumatoid arthritis is either cold or heat therapy. Although both heat and cold are effective, patients who use cold therapy experience almost two times the pain relief as those who use the heat therapy. The majority prefer heat therapy, however, because the cold seems uncomfortable when the ice pack is first applied. But cold therapy offers more benefits in the length of sleep of patients, the number of oral analgesics they need to take and the degree of swelling.

For hands and feet a hot and cold water soak twice a day is helpful. Add two tablespoons of Epsom salts to the water. For a cold pack, mix six ice cubes with a quart of tap water in an 11 inch by 13 inch plastic bag. Place the bag on the inflamed joint for twenty minutes three times a day. For the heat pack, heat a water bottle to 130 degrees Fahrenheit or use a heating pad that goes to a temperature of approximately 130 degrees. Apply for twenty minutes three times a day.

I've heard of a remarkable oil that helps mightily in relieving arthritic pain. It makes aching joints mobile again, so I'm told. It's called *Nature's Oils Plus*. It contains all sorts of wonderful ingredients, including Norwegian cod liver oil. There isn't a thing unnatural about it. Every ingredient is made by God, not man — such as emulsified EPA, DHA, GLA — formulated in a remarkable base that is extracts and essential oils. It can be ordered from Swanson's Health Products. (Address elsewhere.)

Available at your health store also is a pain relieving skin cream called *Camocare*. It's principal ingredient is chamomile, famous as an herbal tea and as a pain suppressant. It's reputed to bring relief to arthritis and muscle pain. And of course, there's the good old standby Ben Gay, which millions swear by. It contains ingredients to reduce inflammation, so use it freely.

The FDA has recently approved of a new drug named

Voltaren. It's being widely hailed as the most effective new weapon against arthritis. It is supposed to have few side effects. Ask your doctor about it. If it's simply another anti-inflammatory drug — such as Motrin, Feldene and Clinoril — it will not cure, but it *will* provide relief from the pain. For those who cannot take such anti-inflammatory medications because of stomach distress, there are rectal suppositories of the same medications. Effective, too, is physical therapy including ultrasound, ice pack or heat. An exercise program, such as walking, biking, swimming or yoga is essential to keep the muscles mobile. Avoid high level aerobics, they're too stimulating. Stay with low level.

The drug *Methotrexate* is an anti-cancer drug which is unexpectedly effective against rheumatoid arthritis. It's a major drug for treating several types of cancer. In lower dosages it is proving a powerful weapon in treating rheumatoid arthritis. Ask your doctor about it — but have him read the side effects to you. Another new drug which has recently been approved for sale here in America is *Flurbiprofen*. It is said to give the same relief as aspirin and ibuprofen with lower doses. It will be sold under the brand name of *Ansaid*.

Ancient Chinese Massage — You can learn how to use 5,000-year-old acupressure techniques to relieve the pain of arthritis that are safe, simple and require only two 15-minutes sessions a day. Michael Reed Gach's book, *Arthritis Relief at Your Fingertips* (Warner) tells you how. Gach has used it on thousands of arthritis sufferers at his Acupressure Institute in Berkeley, California.

Copper Bracelets — If you suffer from arthritic pain or inflammatory conditions, do wear a copper bracelet. If folks laugh at your "superstition," laugh right along with them. You may have the last laugh. I've seen it work wonders.

Sea Mussel — Research with an extract derived from the New Zealand green-lipped mussel is proving to be extremely promising in the treatment of arthritis. Capsules may be ordered from Swanson's, but keep seeking the extract which sooner or later will be available here.

Tea Tree Oil — Mix three to five drops of Tea Tree Oil into a small amount of baby oil or Ben Gay and massage deeply into joints. Or apply it directly to pain areas. It works like magic. Along with a sensible change of diet, it has been known to achieve a total cure. See Chapter 18 for more on Tea Tree Oil. Available at health stores or order from Swanson's.

The Arthritis Foundation has established a "hot line" for arthritics to call regarding the latest information to aid patients. See the last chapter for the toll-free number.

Backaches

Backache seems to be a universal complaint. I've gathered some ideas which may help prevent problems or aid those you may be already experiencing.

1) *Increase vitamin* C — Chronic disk sufferers can be aided tremendously and perhaps avoid surgery. Take from 750 mg to more than 2000 mg a day to help maintain tissues, ligaments, tendons, joints and muscles. Start with small doses and gradually increase. Should diarrhea occur, lower your intake.

2) *Use a Lapboard* — Those who work at desks are constantly admonished not to bend forward. But how can you do desk work without bending forward? I solved the problem! I write constantly on books or home study lessons for publication. I found "bending forward" to be quite agonizing. So I had a lap board made with a rounded cut-out for

my tummy. I prop the board on the arms of my desk chair and on the front edge of my desk. Using it for a slanted writing board, I lean back in my chair and write by the hour. I always make sure to get up and walk around occasionally. I stretch my arms, flex my shoulders, drop over at the waist and bounce my upper torso up and down, flexing the back. It's the pause that refreshes.

3) *Chairs — Chairs!* — Do select your favorite chairs carefully, your desk chair and your TV chair. First, the desk chair. Make sure the seat extends to fit behind the knees when you sit up straight, assuring that your thighs will be parallel to the floor. Your feet should rest flat on the floor. The chair should be firm. It should not slant backward. Your spine should be supported in an erect position. You may need a small soft pillow at the small of your back. Or purchase one of those spinal cushions which are structured to support the lower back during long periods of sitting. As to your typing chair, I can't advise, but I'd think the same applies. Your TV chair shouldn't be totally soft — not enough for your back to sag. It should offer firm support. If you tilt back with your feet raised, find a chair that will allow your feet to be supported. Many such chairs leave the feet hanging in the air. You may need to add a small soft pillow behind your head so your neck isn't strained to view the television. I use a soft "rolled" pillow that fits easily into my neck curve, probably available from *Comfortably Yours*. If you tend to go to sleep easily, do purchase one of those neck pillows that fit snugly around the back of the neck so that your neck and head are supported. Otherwise you'll wake up with a painful neck. Also available from *Comfortably Yours* or other "medical" catalogs.

4) *The Vacuum Cleaner!* — The bane of housework!

There's the upright and there's the canister type. Most uprights require a bent back, at just the right angle to create a "catch" between the shoulders. I like the tank type that can be yanked around on wheels, using my arms and legs instead of my back. The light "wand" can be more easily manipulated. To reach the difficult places I actually get down on my knees to avoid the backbend.

5) *Making the Bed* — A close second to vacuuming. Again, get on your knees. Or try keeping the knees straight and bending from the waist. Quite a feat, but better than the catch between the shoulders.

6) *Sleeping* — The mattress should be firm, not hard and not soft. Some put a board directly under the mattress cover to achieve hardness. Such hardness won't let the natural curves relax, but some seem to need it. Sleeping on a palette on the floor has corrected many back problems. A soft mattress can't support the body and it allows the back to sag in the wrong places. Avoid sleeping on your stomach, it causes the back to "sway" and increases muscle stress. When rising from a prone position, turn on your side and push yourself up with your arms. Sitting straight up stresses the lower back.

If you can afford it you may want to order a special mattress pad containing magnets which relieves aching muscles and bones — even arthritis. I use one and there is a very noticeable difference. I highly recommend it. Its magnetic "points" press into meridians throughout the body, stimulating the points and restoring the flow of Ki throughout the body. If interested, contact Ruby M. Morrow. (Address elsewhere)

7) *Reaching* — Keep a kick stepladder in the kitchen to avoid constantly reaching upward. Pots and pans are usually stored lower down, so buy a rack or storage bin to

hold them at waist level so that you can pull it out and avoid all that stooping and bending. Or buy a revolving shelf, if possible. It will save much awkward seeking, lifting and shifting.

8) *Lifting* — Bend the knees and lift with your arms and legs, never the bent back. Don't kick a heavy load forward with one foot. Don't twist at the waist — pivot with your feet instead.

9) *Washing Dishes* — Do buy a plastic bottle with a brush on top to enable you to wash standing erect. Or install a hand held dishwasher. It could save money in the long run. Leaning forward to wash dishes can be *so* uncomfortable. Do buy a throw rug or rubber mat to stand on, but make sure it doesn't slide on your linoleum floor. When loading the dishwasher, try bending the knees instead of your back. Don't bend over too long.

10) *Gravity Bars* — Do buy a gravity bar and hang upside down, but only if you can find one with separate ankle boots. These bars are marvelous for stretching the back, eliminating many backaches and headaches. *But use it only when someone else is present, never when you're alone.* Don't buy one with the ankle boots attached to the frame because the ankle boots could "lock" and need a second person to release them. It's dangerous. You could be "locked in" for hours, even days. Again, don't use it when alone. Some people should never hang in an inverted position. Do check with your doctor before trying one of these bars.

11) *Homeopathic Help* — Try the homeopathic remedy called *Alpha BP.*

12) *Insoles for Support* — See an orthopedic doctor and have shock-absorbing insoles made to be worn in your shoes. They could totally eliminate your back problems. Or buy insoles at shoe or sporting good stores. Good ones

are *Orthex Relievers*, *Viscolas* or *Sorbothane*. If your chiropractor or osteopath tells you your back problem could be because one leg is shorter than the other, he or she may suggest an insole in only one shoe or by building up the shoe's heel and sole.

Spinal Discs — Hail the new *MRI machine!* — a new technique involving a *magnetic resonance imaging* machine. The patient lies inside the machine while magnetic waves are focused upon his/her spinal column and then fed into a computer. The screen then flashes detailed pictures of the spine, much sharper than myelography. The myelograph requires the injection of a dye into the spinal column, which registers on an x-ray photo — and isn't always sharp. It's also often painful and frequently dangerous. Do ask for an *MRI* exam instead of the usual test if you have a disc problem.

Foot Care

It's strange how one takes walking for granted. . . until a foot problem develops and denies that privilege. I know. An inflamed heel prevented my leading an important tour to Egypt in 1987. So I strongly encourage care of the feet. I offer these suggestions to help:

Select a low-heeled lace-up walking shoe rather than a slip-on if you have problem feet. Buy only leather shoes so your feet can breathe. Don't buy plastic shoes or sneakers. The plastic manmade materials and inserted rubber create all manner of foot problems. Wearing sneakers or tennis shoes can cause cancer from the chemicals contained in them.

When showering or tub bathing, always scrub your feet with a soap bath. Thoroughly dry them, especially between the toes. Then rub a good foot cream into them — castor oil is excellent. Trim toenails just after a tub soak, straight across the top to prevent ingrown toenails. If you already have ingrown toenails, push cotton into and under the toenail of the big toe after trimming, until the nail has grown out long enough to cut straight across the top. Always wear cotton or wool socks. Never wear shoes or even slippers without protective socks or hose. Never, never wear high heels. To do so guarantees trouble with the spine, difficulty in childbirth, trouble with the feet, and trouble with health in general. (Some women declare they *must* occasionally wear high heels for comfort! To each his own.)

Do soak your feet in a foot bath occasionally. The best method is to soak first in hot water for three minutes, then plunge them into cold for one minute. Repeat several times. Finish with the cold. If time prevents soaking, do stand in the bathtub and place your feet under running water, alternating between hot and cold.

Be sure to buy a proper shoe size and, equally important, be sure socks and hosiery are not too small. Many foot problems result from ill-fitting footwear. When shopping for shoes, choose late day hours when the feet are expanded from activity. Purchasing shoes when the feet are not so expanded can result in a bad fit.

Do use the hours watching TV to apply reflexology and massage to your feet. Study a good book on reflexology and apply pressure to the effective points for better health. Do the same to points on your hands.

Heel Pain — At the first sign of a problem see a podiatrist. My podiatrist made plaster casts of both my feet, from which were made plastic insoles to wear in my shoes. They hold my feet in balance. Otherwise, my feet turn inward at the ankle, throwing strain upon the arch. I wear them even now in all my walking shoes. In other shoes I wear Dr. Scholl's soft insoles or *Luxis* shoe supports. Plus I wear a heel pad in one shoe because one leg is shorter than the other. The Luxis inserts can be ordered from Luxis International (address elsewhere).

My heel pain seemed to come from small individual hard crystallized deposits forming a horseshoe around the back of my heel, underneath, plus a hard deposit in the center of each heel. To break them up, I used the erasure end of a pencil probing deeply into them. I applied a good vibrator. A foot Jacuzzi at my doctor's office also helped. Also, my dedicated chiropractor used his strong thumbs to "dig into" the deposits, breaking them up.

If possible, buy a home "spa" to be placed in your tub bath. Let the swirling water focus on your heels. It seems to help break up crystallized deposits. I also used Ben Gay with Tea Tree Oil added on my heels. It seems to heal the inflammation. And castor oil proved to be extremely effective. Using it persistently may have been one reason my heels improved. Wear heel pads in your shoes if it helps. Soft insoles are a great help — they cushion the impact of walking.

Heel pain is now believed to be caused by tiny stress fractures, not calcium deposits called "bone spurs." There are now special x-rays, such as bone scans and tomography (varying "depth" x-rays) enabling doctors to make a more thorough diagnosis. It no longer seems advisable to have surgery to remove spurs, since apparently they are not the cause of your pain. To aid stress fractures researchers advise stretching the back of your ankles to release tight lower leg muscles. Try this for stretching calves and back of ankles: Stand a few feet from a table. Lean forward to grip the edge of the table. Bring one foot forward, bending the knee. Keep the other knee straight. Lean forward, stretching the back of the straight leg. Alternate legs.

Gout — Take the following formula three times daily until the pain subsides. Two teaspoons of apple cider vinegar mixed with 2 teaspoons of raw honey and 1/4 teaspoon tincture of lobelia in a cup of distilled water. This formula should quickly dissipate the excessive uric acid. Temporarily avoid all meat and meat products, eating only salads and soups. Meat is the greatest carrier of uric acid and urea. So said Dr. Som.

Headaches

There is now available a neck collar containing a cold gel which, placed around the neck, often relieves headaches. There's also available a "cold hat" which consists of a cap like a shower cap. It contains a liner filled with a material which freezes yet stays soft and pliable. Placed over the head at the first symptom of a headache it can bring considerable relief. Instead of an ice pack try a package of frozen peas for headache pain. It conforms to the contour of the body better than an ice pack. The cold constricts swollen blood vessels and helps eliminate pain.

Also available is an object called *Choju* which is an electronic acupuncture device without needles. By pushing a button on the end of the device it generates small pulses of electricity which stimulates the pain area to reduce the pain. Its theory is that, applied to acupuncture points, it balances the meridians allowing life force to flow through to relieve pain. It can be used not only for headaches but all over the body except near the eyes. It should also be used only under the direction of a physician because it can affect heart patients and pregnant women. It should not be used on infants. It's available from Swanson.

A remarkable new nose spray known as *DHE 45* works within one to three hours to relieve migraine headaches. It's superior to oral drugs or injections. It can be used anywhere. Relief can last for days or weeks. The side effects are slight — nasal congestion in a few and a bitter taste in even fewer.

Apply Tea Tree Oil to painful areas. Mix it with Ben Gay if you wish. Apply Olbas Oil or White Flower Oil in each nostril and inhale deeply. Or try the homeopathic remedy called *Gelsemmium*. And try an herbal capsule called *Feverfew*. Take one capsule daily to avoid tensions that cause headaches, especially migraines. For a migraine headache try putting your thumb against the inside palate of your upper mouth and press.

Both migraine and cluster headaches are believed to be caused by allergies to some foods and/or food additives. Nitrates, nitrites (found in prepared and preserved foods) and chocolate are just a few found to be the offenders in some people. So you may want to experiment with the foods you eat, like cold cuts, for example. Bologna and all cold cuts definitely cause headache. Avoid! They contain both nitrates and nitrites which dilate blood vessels.

Millions of Americans wind up in hospital emergency rooms each year seeking the only real relief from an agonizingly severe headache — a narcotic drug. But take heart, migraine sufferers, because there is a new drug treatment that is highly effective and *nonnarcotic*. This new drug, *Intravenous Prochlorperazine*, has no serious side effects and no danger of addiction, as the narcotics do.

Do choose one of those cervical pillows that are made to fit the curve of your neck and throat. I've already suggested a special chiropractor's or osteopath's pillow — order from Dr. Noll Walker if unavailable locally (see Chapter 20). It's amazing how fewer headaches I have since purchasing one from him. The "roll" on one side accommodates the normal person with the normal neck length. The "roll" on the other side accommodates the petite person with small bones and neck — like me.

Exercises For Headaches

1) Sit on a stool. First stretch your arms above your head. Now lock the hands low down behind the head. Inhale. Exhale, bending forward to let your head hang between the knees. With your clasped hands, pull your head down and down. Stretch, stretch your neck down with a bouncing action, turning the head from side to side. Repeat 3 times.

2) Either standing, or lying on your back, inhale, turn your head slowly to line up your chin with your right shoulder. Gently stretch the chin back further, hold, then return to center and exhale. Repeat on left side. Gentle stretches on both sides.

Hip Pain — An amazing natural home remedy will help those with a "problem" hip — aching in the hip joints. A doctor from India gave me the following remedy: from your backyard, gather enough soil to make a small poultice. Placing foil under it, moisten the soil and place in your oven for ten minutes at about 300 degrees. Wrap the foil and soil with a towel, place it on the hip, removing layers of the towel as the compress cools. Dry heat or moist heat may be applied. One may sit on this poultice while watching television prior to bed or one can apply it directly to the hip during sleep. Repeating this routine several times a week for about three weeks should heal the hip.

Or you may wish to make a poultice of crushed comfrey instead of the soil and apply it to your aching spine or a problem hip. You may also wish to add fresh comfrey to the soil pack or alternate between it and the fresh comfrey pack.

Osteoporosis — This is a medical term for bone loss. It occurs in women more than men. Here are some helpful suggestions:

1) Do take silica and magnesium tablets even now, if you're over 35. Take silica rather than calcium. And take as much or more magnesium than silica. To repeat, it's lack of silica, even more than calcium, which causes bone loss.

2) Do take estrogen (women) after menopause if your doctor advises. Take it only on your doctor's advice. But take the lowest possible dosage, the green or brown pills, called *Premarin*, or the tablet called *Estriol*, which is usually carried only by holistic doctors. And insist that progesterone be given along with the estrogen therapy. Otherwise you could become a candidate for uterus cancer. Estrogen-Progesterone therapy or Estriol helps avoid hip or spine fractures. Avoid the cheaper generic estrogen pills. They are often synthetic. They often cause bloating and make the tummy and hips "fatter." But see my section on estrogen and realize you *must* also take progesterone to balance the estrogen intake. Silica-magnesium should be taken with minor doses of estrogen to enhance the calcium in the silica.

Brittle Bones — As one grows older the bones grow brittle. This means they have become porous with large hollow tubes or canals running through them — long open spaces that should be mineralized or filled with mineral deposits. The major cause of demineralized or brittle bones is inactivity. You simply haven't been exercising enough. The first thing you must do is begin taking walks, or walk-in-place. Do some form of regular exercise. Do back-bends or forward bends to flex the spine. Such activity keeps minerals flowing into the bones. When you remain too inactive the minerals simply seep out of your bony structure.

Try yogic exercise. The first to attempt is walking on your hands and knees, gently at first. Then increase your pace until you are actually running around on them. To make the exercise doubly effective, try diaphragmatic breathing at the same time. Pant like a dog — short panting breaths with the lips closed. When this panting is done, sitting in yoga posture we call it the "breath of fire." Repeat the panting exercise standing before an open window as you are retiring. This oxygenizes the blood and results in better relaxation and sleep.

Brittle bones also indicate a lack of calcium-magnesium and silica, probably for many years. The latest research indicates silica to be the best form of calcium — much superior to calcium tablets, which can cause arthritis. Buy silica and magnesium capsules at your health store. Lack of silica causes not only brittle bones but broken fingernails and thinning hair. Don't take bone meal tablets for calcium. They contain lead. If you insist on taking calcium rather than silica, be aware that you do not need it in abundance. It is better to under-take than over-take. Moderation is the key word. Always take magnesium with calcium.

Brittle bones usually appear in geriatric cases. Older persons seem to lose their supply of calcium-magnesium and silica. Falls often result in fractured hips, or other bones, which can lead to pneumonia. In elderly people this can often be fatal. Elderly people should certainly be taking a daily supply of magnesium tablets and silica. Should bones be broken, add vitamin C, D and E to the diet. They aid in healing broken bones.

According to Dr. Guy E. Abraham, former professor of Gynecologic Endocrinology at the UCLA Medical School, one should take twice as much magnesium as calcium. He states, "If the government reversed the daily requirements for calcium and magnesium you could clear out the hospitals in 5 years." He feels the imbalance of calcium and magnesium causes premature aging, arthritis, allergies, heart disease, kidney stones and senility.

He feels that if you want to slow the aging process, start taking twice as much magnesium as you take calcium. The late Dr. Hans Selye, a Nobel Laureate in Physiology and Medicine, agreed. In his book *Calciphylaxis*, he states that magnesium intake should certainly equal the intake of calcium. Well, many doctors are beginning to agree. It's certainly worth trying. My own opinion is that it's the calcium in pasteurized milk that creates havoc. It isn't balanced by magnesium.

Pain Relief

Do try *Nutra-Cell Anti-Pain* tablets which consist of aspirin buffered with magnagel and DLPA, unless you are allergic to aspirin. Available at your health store or from Swanson's catalog. Apparently if you take this tablet daily soon it will vanquish the pain altogether. The DLPA is an amino acid.

Electromagnetic Therapy — is the methodology of the

future. When dis-ease appears in the body it's because certain cells have developed an abnormal behavior pattern. Every cell in the body has a built-in electrical charge. Electric charges from some electrical machines, such as the TENS, can restore balance to the out-of-tune cells, relieving pain and restoring normalcy.

Hot and Cold Therapy — Apply heat to improve blood circulation and to release the tension in knotted muscles. Use cold to reduce blood circulation and act as an anesthetic in treating strains and muscle spasms. Contact a good osteopathic physician or chiropractor who, using a special manipulative technique, can relieve muscle tension and restore balance to the spine. Osteopaths often recommend wearing a support to reduce strain on back muscles. An excellent choice is called the *Levitor.* It's a light five-ounce device that relieves strain on muscles caused by gravity. It very gently and gradually improves the posture and nudges the spine into balance. For full information, contact the Kirksville College of Osteopathic Medicine. (Address elsewhere).

Relieving Muscle Pain — To relieve common muscle pain there are several simple exercises which help. Sit on the floor and grasp your toes. Pull them toward you. Repeat several times. Stand on a step or stair and alternate letting each heel drop below the edge. This is great for stretching the calf muscles. Both these exercises should relieve charley horse. For tennis elbow fill a plastic shopping bag with 7 or 8 pounds of fruit or canned goods. With your forearm flat on the table, palm up, grasp the bag and slowly raise it about 10 times. Repeat morning and night. For neck muscles apply a cold pack — even a package of frozen peas. Cold packs are now available which wrap around the painful area and tie, for 20 minute treatments. For shoulder pain try the homeopathic remedy called *Mag Phos*.

Music and Pain — More than once music has been proven to alleviate pain. Played for terminally ill patients it dramatically relaxes the muscles and reduces stress, anxiety and states of depression. Music therapy has been known to be so effective that analgesics were discontinued. Eight out of ten patients benefit from it. The music should be quiet and calming and the patient should be lying down for the best benefits of relaxation. When the consciousness gets totally involved in the music muscles react by relaxing. Try it in your own home since soothing music cannot harm you in any way. Incidentally, music can also cause tension and illness. Any tempo that is faster than the human heartbeat raises tension and blood pressure. Rock music has been known to kill canaries.

Chapter Thirteen

Colds, Allergies and Viruses

The Germ Theory — It was Pasteur in 1895 who gave birth to the "germ theory" — maintaining that the diseases of mankind were caused by germs and germ bacteria, and the entire medical world embraced his theory, and still does so today. Only a few of the great minds in medical science today believe and understand that a pure, healthy body possesses a natural innate immunity to germs because we live in an ocean of germs, ready to invade any human system that is weakened by pollution, toxins and poisons. Rudolph Virchow vigorously opposed Pasteur's theory. He stated, "If I could live my life over again, I would devote it to proving that germs seek their natural habitat — diseased tissue — rather than being the cause of the diseased tissue."

The holistic physician today fully realizes that microbes and germs are scavengers and can gain a foothold in the body only when there is decay, waste, toxins and pollution. This is the breeding ground for germs and an impure system will be invaded by them. Many new age doctors and researchers believe that *germs are never the cause of a disease*. They are the result of a polluted human system. To submit to all sorts of immunizing programs is not the answer to avoiding disease. The answer is to purify the body through food, drink and exercise, and nature will see to it that the germs and bacteria in the atmosphere do not find a welcome home in your body.

Colds: Prevention and Cure — If the above is true, you can only "catch" a cold if your system is fertile ground for the germs to gain a foothold. The way to prevent a cold is to keep the immune system properly balanced through raw foods, less flesh food, fresh vegetables, fruits, grains, nuts, food supplements, a good attitude and plenty of rest. Oh, yes, and some degree of exercise, even brisk walking.

When you consider that if a room full of people are all exposed to someone with a cold, only a few will "catch" the cold, it must then be true that germs can only hibernate in weakened immune systems. Colds can only establish a foothold when the body's resistance is weak, usually through the intake of improper carbohydrates — products with white sugar, white flour, white salt, processed foods. The first part of the system to be affected is the upper respiratory area. The moment there is warning of a cold, consider the following:

1) Suck slowly on a zinc lozenge. One or two a day.

2) Take vitamin C every hour.

3) Take Propolis capsules, available at health stores* — three with breakfast, three with lunch, three with dinner, three at bedtime.

4) If your throat is sore gargle with Oxyquiniline

* See *The Book of Beginning Again* for details regarding Propolis.

water (three tiny homeopathic sulfur tablets dissolved in 4 oz. of water). Take a mouthful of the water, gargle with it several times, then swallow it. Repeat several times a day. The one glassful should last all day. You should keep Oxyquiniline in your home at all times; it's available from any homeopathic pharmacy. If you have difficulty finding it, order from Standard Homeopathic Pharmacy (address elsewhere). The sulfate (pure sulfur powder) will kill infection throughout the body.

5) If you don't have Oxyquiniline tablets for a sore throat, try this: one-half glass apple cider vinegar, one-half glass water, one teaspoon sea salt, Real Salt or any good mineral salt. Mix these ingredients. Take a large mouthful of the liquid and gargle, pause, gargle, pause and gargle many times with the same mouthful. (Don't swallow it.) Repeat in an hour or two. The glassful should last the entire day. Gargle with one mouthful at a time. If too strong, add more water.

Another excellent remedy for sore throat is Tea Tree Oil. Add three to six drops of the oil (make sure it is pure Tea Tree Oil) to warm water and gargle with it. Or add three drops of the pure oil to half a glass of juice or lemonade and sip slowly.

6) Take echinacea herb tablets to boost the immune system and fight infection. Or take garlic tablets. Or both.

7) Go to bed and rest

8) Drink plenty of water (consider *purified* water) and juices. You must have fluids, up to 8 glasses a day. Avoid iced liquids. They will further irritate not only your throat but your stomach as well.

9) If there is congestion, try this: to one-half glass of grapefruit juice, add one-half glass of hot water. Mix six drops of oil of eucalyptus with one-half teaspoon of sugar.

Put the sugar in your mouth and drink it down with the glass of grapefruit juice.

Again, pure Tea Tree Oil to the rescue for congestion, too. Rub the pure oil onto the chest and back. Add a bit to your steam vaporizer and inhale. Sprinkle some on your pillow before sleeping.

Or try Cayce's Campho-Derm on the chest and the soles of the feet for congestion. Yes, feet!

10) Avoid any product containing *phenylpropanolamine*, or *PPA*, a drug often used in over-the-counter cold medicines, diet preparations, and aids for sleeping. It's extremely dangerous. It can cause a stroke by triggering a sharp rise in blood pressure — especially if it's followed by caffeine. So says the journal of the AMA. This isn't the same as *phenylalanine*, an amino acid which is good for you. So don't get them confused.

11) If you lose your sense of taste or smell after a cold, try *zinc* compounds.

12) To ease cold symptoms try drinking a full glass of water with 10 or 20 drops of red-hot chili sauce in it once a day. Or take *cayenne* herb tablets.

13) Suck wild cherry or honey lozenges from the health store — they soothe the throat. Avoid menthol, minted or medicated drops or lozenges. They dry and irritate an already inflamed throat.

14) Before buying a drug store product for your cough, first try the health store for a honey-lemon concoction. Or make your own.

15) Prepare a concoction of: one-half glass of ginger water, one-half glass of raw milk, one teaspoon of raw honey. Drink it hot and stay covered up warmly. To make the ginger water: break off about 2 inches of ginger from the ginger root; add it to one cup of water; boil down to 1/2

cup of water. Add the raw milk and the honey. This ginger-milk drink at bedtime could get you through the cold or flu season with no problems.

16) If you are "into" the Edgar Cayce products, order from wherever Cayce products are sold: *Glyco-thymoline* for gargling; *Vapohaler* as an inhalant and decongestant, for hay fever, sinusitis; *Insprol* for asthma, bronchitis, coughs, colds; *Campho-Derm* as a liniment to rub on the chest and feet for a cold and to rub over the kidneys for kidney complaints. And don't forget the castor oil pack for just about everything.

How to Overcome the Flu — From a health store buy: a bottle of echinacea herb capsules; a bottle of chaparral herb capsules; a bottle of strong vitamin C; a bottle of Propolis capsules; a bottle of blackstrap molasses; a package of flowers of sulfur or a bottle of Oxyquiniline; a package of red root herb powder; a package of bayberry bark herb powder; a bottle of cranberry juice; a bottle of aspirin; a bottle of garlic capsules; a bottle of papaya juice; a bottle of vegetable juice.

Go to bed. Stay warm. Stop eating and begin drinking water and juices. The cranberry juice prevents the virus from entering the bladder and urinary tract. Every two hours alternate between two echinacea herb capsules and chaparral. On the hour in between take from one to three vitamin C tablets and from one to three Propolis capsules, and a garlic capsule. Thus, for example; 8 a.m. — two echinacea; 9 a.m. — vitamin C, Propolis and garlic; 10 a.m. — two chaparral; 11 a.m. — vitamin C, Propolis and garlic. Continue this through the day. Have someone make tea at least twice a day with the red root herb powder combined with the bayberry herb powder. The tea isn't essential but it helps.

Mix 3 tablespoons of blackstrap molasses with one tablespoon of sulfur powder. Take one teaspoon in the morning and another at night. Gargle with Oxyquiniline (a sulfur tablet) if your throat is sore. I've just said to dissolve 3 tiny tablets in 4 oz. of water. Order both sulfur powder and Oxyquiniline sulfur tablets from Standard Homeopathic Pharmacy. (Address elsewhere)

Should you feel hungry drink a glass of juice. Alternate between cranberry, papaya, vegetable or fresh citrus juice. If you fail to have bowel elimination either take an enema once a day or take a natural herbal laxative, such as psyllium or flaxseed. Drink plenty of water, rest. Take aspirin. Aspirin seems to contain a healing quality as well as that of pain control. But most need the herbal treatment for complete recovery. If you *must* eat try soup.

Try the homeopathic remedy called *Gelsemmium*.

Take flu injections at your own risk. My mother never had flu till her doctor persuaded her she needed a flu shot every fall as a routine. She had flu and a dreadful cold every winter after that and was in bed weeks at a time, till I persuaded her to stop the injections. Maybe they help some people, but I personally wouldn't take them. However, I know a few elderly people who swear by them and take them every year. So use your own judgment. Many who take them promptly come down with flu.

Write Hanna Kroeger, (address elsewhere), and inquire how to avoid the flu. She may offer special products as good or better than those I've suggested. Her Anti-Flu herb tablets may work just as well as the flu injections to help you avoid the flu. Michael Tierra will also have a marvelous herbal prevention and cure. The flu strain these days is a powerful virus. But every doctor I know admits antibiotics will neither prevent it or help you recover from it. But there may be other drugs which are effective if the above program fails to heal you.

Sinus Congestion — We healthians would rather not take Dristan, Contact, etc. because of the chemical and artificial ingredients as well as the side affects. So we constantly seek help from more natural products. Such a product seems to be *Sinus-ade*. Its distributors claim it to be a natural nasal decongestant which restores natural breathing and aids hay fever, allergies, colds and flu. Just a suggestion. Probably available from Swanson's Health Products (Address elsewhere). But the daily use of a Neti Pot is much to be preferred. Also try *Cobiozin* from your health store. Later, I will tell you how to use the Neti Pot and where one can be purchased.

Home remedies include taking vitamin C daily or try *Propolis*. Obtain both from your health store. You can take both daily forever with only good effects. Use pure *Tea Tree Oil* in a steam vaporizer. Rub drops around sinuses. *Olbas oil* is good. *White Flower Herbal Oil* is great. (Available from the Trace Co., address elsewhere.) Or *eucalyptus* — rub on the end of your nose and insert a drop with a fingertip up each nostril and inhale. Adding vitamin B6 to the diet can also aid in overcoming sinus problems. Take *goldenseal herb capsules*, three a day. Within a few days the impacted sinuses should begin to drain.

If you insist, try antihistamines such as *Benadryl*. It will make you sleepy. Try *Terfenadine* or *Hismanal*, which will *not* make you sleepy. But don't stay on them. They are *not* good for you. Be cautious with decongestants if you have high blood pressure or an irregular heartbeat. Use these products only as long as absolutely necessary. Propolis from the health store is much to be preferred. Drug store decongestants should be taken only if your doctor approves.

If you exercise daily your own body will produce natural adrenaline from stimulated adrenal glands. If you can't exercise then do the *yogic cobra pose* — which is to lie face down on the floor, raise the upper torso with your arms, arching your back and tilting the head back. It's like a backbend lying down. Support your upper torso with your arms. Hold the pose as long as comfortable. The cobra pose is also excellent for stimulating the adrenal glands. (See Chapter 14 under *Fatigue and the Adrenal Glands*.)

Change the filter in your air conditioner at least once a season. Filter replacements are inexpensive and easy to install. Air conditioning systems can keep the air you breathe cleaner if the filter works properly.

If you have a chronic sinus infection check for an infected tooth or a deep-down problem with your eyes. Not very plausible but very possible. Consider removing dental silver fillings.

To open the sinuses place the thumb on the cheek bone and slide it downward under the cheekbone so that you are able to lift upward on the bone. With small lifts work your way toward the spot where the cheekbone joins with the nose. You may find the spot extremely painful, especially if your sinuses are plugged. Here you will press upward, lifting the cheekbone. You not only are opening the maxillary sinuses but you are stimulating an important acupuncture point. Release the upward lift and repeat it several times — at the juncture where the cheekbone joins the nose. With the thumb and forefinger spread the wings of the nose wide apart and sniff rapidly in and out. There should be no further obstruction. If you have problems breathing because of adenoids sleep on the left side, if possible.

Or try the following to begin drainage: either standing or sitting upright, slowly, slowly tip the head backwards until you are gazing directly at the ceiling. Slowly try to touch your nose with your lower lip. Repeat for a slow count of fifty. Drainage of the sinuses should begin about halfway through the maneuver. This exercise was suggested by Doctors Gladys and William McGarey of the A.R.E. Clinic in Phoenix, Arizona. Write them for further advice or for ordering Edgar Cayce health products. Send your inquiry to Cayce Corner (address elsewhere).

Neti Pot and Well-Being — To aid in colds or sinus problems and for general well-being do this ancient Indian method of purification. Prepare a water and salt solution by this method: Into one quart of water place 1/4 cup of sea salt or Real Salt. Bring it to a boil and boil for five minutes. Allow it to cool, then store in an airtight container. During your shower, fill a nasal douche or Neti Pot with this salt water. Tilt your head to the right, insert the nozzle of the Neti Pot into the left nostril. Let the salt solution flow into your left nostril and out the right. Keep the mouth open. If any enters the throat, eject the solution through your mouth. Repeat through the right nostril. Do not swallow.

If you cannot find a nasal douche to purchase order a Neti Pot from the Himalayan International Institute (address elsewhere). Daily use of the Neti Pot could change your whole health picture. If you haven't a supply of the prepared salt water available, or if you wish to practice it outside the shower, fill the Neti Pot with lukewarm water with one scant teaspoon of salt. Make very sure the salt is completely dissolved in the water. Lean over the bathroom lavatory and proceed to cleanse each nostril as described above. Then close one nostril and blow forcibly, then reverse. Now, closing each nostril with the thumb, breathe in and out vigorously to remove remaining moisture. Then blow through both nostrils simultaneously. Lean over for a moment to allow more moisture to drain.

Neti not only controls sinus problems, but it also controls headaches, sinus congestion, eliminates colds, eye problems, tonsillitis, depression, asthma, bronchitis and aids insomnia, and epilepsy. Caution: make sure water isn't too hot; don't remove moisture too forcibly; make sure salt is dissolved; don't use if you suffer from chronic nose bleeds.

Nose Sprays — Nasal sprays account for a large percentage of chronic or long-standing nasal congestion. Those who habitually are congested may be causing their own problem because they are addicted to the nose drops they use. The nose drops bring immediate relief because the drugs constrict tiny blood vessels and reduce localized swelling. But once its effectiveness wears off, the dilation of the vessels returns and they become engorged with blood, swelling the tissues beyond their original state. The nose spray addict reaches again for the drops or spray and another cycle of nasal congestion ensues, the addict never once suspecting he may be causing his own congestion.

For a drug-free all natural nasal spray that will not cause addiction, write to the Vermont Country Store for a catalog. Their nasal spray is a saline based, nongreasy gel. (See last chapter for address.)

Allergies — The most common cause of allergies: pollen in the spring. Other allergies include food and cosmetics.

Pollen is the male fertilizing agent of flowering plants. The wind picks it up from the plants and fills the air with it. Millions of people are allergic to this atmospheric pollen. Beginning in February, in the northern hemisphere, most trees begin to pollinate. Summer is the time for ragweed and high concentrations of mold spores. Here are suggestions for help.

1) Again, the Neti Pot. And, again, take bee Propolis, which can be purchased at your health store. This frequently will solve your problem completely. Some are helped by one tablet a day. Others will require three tablets four times a day in order to control the running nose and weeping eyes. Increase or decrease as the need indicates.

2) Keep windows closed at night. Use air conditioners, but make sure their filters are clean. I've already advised concerning humidifiers.

3) Since pollen levels are highest early in the morning, plan your outdoor activities later in the day.

4) Keep your car windows closed.

5) Write your nearest homeopathic pharmacy for their best product for hay fever or allergies. I can suggest *Natura Fed Plus*. Again, try *Cobiozin*, a nondrug natural approach to aid post-nasal drip, sinusitis and allergy, which often simulates a cold; available from your health store. It contains vitamins A, C, B12, pantothenic acid, calcium lactate and zinc gluconate, lemon bioflavonoid complex and thymus, in a base of rose hips, wheat germ, chlorophyll, lymph — which enables the flow of lymph to clear out the sinuses. The thymus produces interferon, which is effective in *all* physical problems.

6) Use only cotton handkerchiefs. Carry them with you always to cover your nose to block out irritating scents. Avoid perfumes which cause the least allergic reactions, such as a drippy nose; avoid scented toilet tissue; always blow your nose through *both* nostrils to avoid sending offending bacteria into the other nostril; remove plastic covers from garments from the cleaners to allow the remaining fumes to escape before wearing; use only cotton

blankets because wool distributes spores which could enter your nostrils; do not use a chemically treated dust cloth.

7) Discard live house plants and use only artificial, unless the dirt molds are covered with sand; don't lap-sit your pets, their fur can cause reactions; don't lie down or bend over during an attack, sit upright with torso slightly forward as if writing at a desk; use acupressure points to relieve pain directly under the eyebrows and under the cheek bones near the nose, as described.

If you take injections for your allergies, a new blood test can determine how well you're responding to treatment, thus eliminating the further need of painful injections. Till now the only gauge of your increased resistance to the allergens was to inject it immediately under the skin, after which you would wait patiently for a reaction. No more. The new test, called the *IgG4FAST* test, requires the doctor to take a small sample of your blood and mix it with a sample of any substance to which you're allergic. Next, the doctor adds another chemical which attaches itself to antibodies your blood has built up against the allergen. The result is a glow. If a bright glow results, it means you are building up enough antibodies so that your system can tolerate that which you've previously reacted to — thus reducing the frequency of injections.

Or ask your doctor to begin giving you small doses of the substances to which you are allergic, then gradually increasing the doses. This encourages your system to build up immunities to the allergens.

Do try the following as an aid against allergies. Into a dropper bottle, pour plain cold pressed castor oil. Drop five drops under your tongue daily. Too simple to be effective? No indeed. The oil builds up the immune system to tolerate many substances not previously tolerated. Try it!

You may want to order castor oil from the Drs. McGarey, just mentioned. Their Cayce product has been cold pressed, which certainly isn't true of drugstore castor oil.

Flowers, Allergies, and Infection — Don't send cut flowers or plants to a sick friend. The water in the vase is a breeding ground for dangerous microorganisms. They could cause infections or allergic reactions. Send artificial flowers! They're gorgeous. You can always touch the petals with rose oil (an essential oil) or some other natural fragrance if you wish. Or send a good book, preferably a joke book — laughter is healing.

Hay Fever — Apply the same instructions as was given for allergies — especially concerning Propolis. Hay fever often resembles a cold. With hay fever nasal discharge is clear. With a cold it's discolored and thick. Be sure your lawn is mowed at least twice a week. Put a plastic cover over your mattress, box springs and pillows, and keep them dusted. Sleep with your windows closed.

Again, try Natura Fed Plus. Its ingredients include Chinese herbal combinations (minor blue dragon) and I'm told the product is quite effective. It may be available at your health store. Also I've heard of a new eye drop that seems to be highly effective for irritated or inflamed eyes and as an aid to hay fever symptoms. It's call *Similasan Drops*. Do seek more information at your health store.

Also, there's a new drug called *Cromalyn* which researchers are hailing. Cromalyn prevents the body from producing histamine which triggers allergic reactions. It's marketed as an inhaler.

If your nose is forever dripping don't be too quick to blame it on pollen or pets. Consider food. The worst offenders are: cheese, milk, eggs, white bread, peanuts, chocolate, beer, wine, shrimp and spices. Milk is especially suspect.

Try buying raw whole milk before you give up on all milk. Also consider that it may be your cosmetics. See *Forever Young* for details.

Vaccinations — Eleanor McBean, long a fighter against enforced vaccination, when all school children are forced to accept vaccination or be banned from school, writes:

"Compulsory vaccination is illegal and you do not have to submit to this disease-producing practice. Any school which requires vaccinations of any kind is violating the law of U.S. and human rights. An example is Bill A.B.1940 of California, which states:

'3384. Immunization of a person shall not be required for admission to a public or private elementary or secondary school if the parent or guardian (in the case of a minor), or the person seeking admission (if an adult) files with the governing board of the school district or the governing authority of the private school, as the case may be, a letter stating that such immunization is contrary to his or her beliefs. However, when there is good cause to believe that a person is suffering from poliomyelitis, the person may be temporarily excluded from the school until the governing board of the school district or the governing authority of the private school is satisfied that the disease does not exist.'"

Parents who do not want their children vaccinated must write a letter to the school principal stating their objections. It need not be a religious reason. It is enough that it is against the wishes or beliefs of the parents.

Puncturing the skin and injecting any foreign substance (as a vaccine) is termed an *operation*, the performance of which constitutes malpractice if given without the willing consent of those involved, says Dr. McBean. But oral vaccination, under force, is equally objectionable.

Here is a polio exemption letter for California residents:

"Date: ______________________

In accordance with the provision of Section 3384, Division 4, of the Health and Safety Code, Chapter 7, under the title "Immunization Against Poliomyelitis," I hereby declare that as a parent (or guardian), in control or charge of ____(child's name)____, a minor enrolled in school, I withhold my consent and request that said minor be exempt from any such vaccination or immunization against polio on the grounds that such is contrary to my beliefs.

Signed ____________________________________
(parent or guardian)
Address ___________________________________"

(Check the statutes in your state to make sure this letter is legal.)

Dr. McBean also states that her research proves that retained vaccine poisons have developed cancers in millions of children. She has seen cancers on the arms, exactly where the vaccine was injected, a few years after the injection. And other diseases, such as encephalitis (brain damage), paralysis (sometimes within 24 hours, but usually later), blindness, open sores, tuberculosis, heart trouble, kidney disease, and death — sometimes instantly and sometimes within a few hours. For further information concerning either needle or oral vaccinations write to: The Better Life Research Foundation, P.O. Box 42002, Los Angeles, California 90042. Or write to Hanna Kroeger for information. Her only child, a daughter, was permanently injured through such vaccinations. She can advise you how to legally prevent such an enforced practice. See last chapter for her address.

Just as an added thought: when Sita, our daughter, was a school child we wrote such a letter of protest to her school principal. She was the only child in her school exempted from vaccination. Every state has an exemption law, but it's like pulling teeth to find out about it. It's kept very quiet. But *do* inquire. If you're unable to locate such a law in your state, just write a letter of protest to your child's school. Or write a document requiring the doctor or nurse administering the vaccine to sign an affidavit guaranteeing the safety of the immunization, and accepting full responsibility for any effect the vaccine has upon the health of the child. That should prevent any enforcement. Even with such a signature, refuse the immunization, even if you have to state "religious reasons." No human being should be forced to put into his/her body any substance to which objections are made.

Phillip Emmerling of Colorado Springs, Colorado, took his three-month-old daughter for her oral polio vaccine in December, 1986. Twenty days later *he* was paralyzed. He is suing the vaccine's maker for $3.25 million.

Mr. Emmerling's attorney, Walter Kyle, states that "the leading cause of polio in this country today is the live polio vaccine." He has worked on six similar cases in the past ten years. He further states: "You can catch the virus from changing diapers or kissing the baby after the child is vaccinated. This has been documented by scientists, but barely mentioned to the public." A spokesman for Lederle Laboratories, manufacturer of the vaccine, refused to comment on the Emmerling case.

Now comes word that Dr. Albert Sabin, the man who "wiped out polio" with an oral vaccine, is now about to eliminate measles with an aerosol vaccine. But no one seems to be aware of or care how these vaccines affect the system later in life. Strange, but Dr. Sabin himself suffered from a mysterious near-fatal paralysis which immobilized his body for many months. According to the report, no cause was ever found. Could it be he took his own vaccines for polio and measles? Whereas such vaccines may "wipe out" polio, could they really be responsible for many other afflictions just as bad, masquerading under a new or different name? — such as multiple sclerosis? — and Parkinson's? — and all the other devastating afflictions for which there is no "known" cause?

Chapter Fourteen

Nervousness and Stress

Nerves, Nervousness, Insomnia — Herbs known to relax the nerves are passiflora, hops, catnip, skullcap, valerian, chamomile, red clover, and lobelia. Lobelia should be combined with any of the others and taken only in small amounts, perhaps 1/4 teaspoon. Those with a nerve disorder should also consider taking a B-complex tincture under the tongue and calcium lactate or calcium gluconate. It is also well to seek the cause of stress.

Tranquilizers — If you need a tranquilizer for anti-anxiety, do ask your doctor about a drug called *Bu-Spar*. It's supposed to be nonaddictive. Others, such as Valium, Atavan, Librium, are addictive.

Valium is the nation's most widely prescribed tranquilizing drug, yet tests have shown that it causes the very symptoms it is supposed to relieve. Doctors prescribe it when there are signs of tension, acute hyperexcited states, anxiety, muscle spasm, fatigue, apprehension, depression, and insomnia, even though they well know the side effects, which are: acute hyperexcited state, anxiety, increased muscle spasticity, drowsiness and fatigue. Thus the patient is given a drug to tranquilize him which will eventually result in the same symptoms from which he seeks relief. In addition, the drug causes liver and kidney damage, resulting in jaundice, and a decrease in the white blood count. And it is addictive. Before prescribing the drug, the patient should be told of the possible side effects. Do try the above herbal remedies before submitting to drug therapy.

Insomnia — Avoid medical tranquilizers in favor of natural herbs and homeopathic remedies such as Calms Forte, Kalms Cap, Silent Night, Good Night, Relaxa-Plex, Coffea. Hanna Kroeger distributes an herbal tea for insomnia. So does Michael Tierra.

Over-the-counter sleeping pills are often more dangerous than prescription pills. They trigger strange side effects, such as blurred or double vision, disorientation, ringing in the ears, dizziness and poor coordination. Take them with great caution. They usually contain antihistamine. Practice the Sanford Bennett exercises of tensing every muscle in the body and then totally relaxing. Do this lying abed. Just before going to bed, step to the window and flap the arms, doing deep breathing exercises simultaneously. Fling the arms backward, inhaling deeply, and forward, exhaling deeply. Repeat several times. This oxygenizes the blood and improves sleep.

Never drink alcohol just before retiring. It can disturb your sleep. When you finally close your eyes, turn your problems over to your subconscious mind, ask it to help you enter a deep, sweet sleep. Focus your attention on your breath rather than your problems. Stop reliving your daily incidents, "If I had it to do again, I'd say ...." Instead, concentrate on your breath.

The common passion flower herb (Passiflora incarnata) may be our best tranquilizer yet, according to University of California ethnobotanist Michael Weiner. The herb both induces a natural sleep and calms hyperactive people. Weiner believes physicians should recommend this plant to patients who want to wean themselves from synthetic sleeping pills and tranquilizers.

Surprisingly, one variety of passion flower was recently found to contain serotonin (P. quandrangularis or Giant Granadilla), a substance produced in the human brain. Patients with chronic depression have been found to have low levels of serotonin in their cerebrospinal fluid. Researchers speculate that adding it to circulating blood would relieve the depression. Weiner theorizes that passion flower acts as a natural calming agent by promoting the transmission of subtle nerve impulses. It appears to aid concentration, alter perception and gently shift mood. Passion flower has no known toxicity in small doses. Weiner says he often brews himself a cup of passion flower at night, using only 1/2 teaspoon of the aromatic herb.

A paper by David R. Hawkins, M.D., of the North Nassau Mental Health Center, New York, establishes startling parallels between tranquilizers and the effects of niacinamide on the brain. A research group from Hoffman-La Roche of Switzerland found that the vitamin has properties in common with certain tranquilizers and barbiturates in regard to effect on spinal cord activity as well as anticonflict, anticonvulsant, antiaggressive, muscle relaxant and hypnotic actions. In fact, the group compares the vitamin's effectiveness with that of a highly potent type of tranquilizer. Do try it also for insomnia. Combine it with herbal capsules mentioned earlier: valerian, etc.

Do consider the following for insomnia:

1) go to bed at the same time and get up at the same time daily;

2) do some deep breathing exercises at bedtime. They relax rather than stimulate taut muscles, and tire the body;

3) take your calcium-magnesium (or silica) capsules at bedtime. They relax you. Also take B6 if you experience muscle cramps in legs or toes during the night;

4) don't eat spicy food for dinner. It could cause digestive problems during the night;

5) don't drink coffee, tea, colas or alcohol after lunch time (preferably never);

6) avoid sleeping pills. Take herb capsules instead, and take herbal tinctures under the tongue. Drink warm raw whole milk at bedtime with a teaspoon of raw honey. The milk contains natural L-Tryptophane, an amino acid that induces the flow of serotonin in the brain, which is known to reduce anxiety and induce sleep. (Avoid L-Tryptophane supplements.)

7) set an alarm clock so you're not worried about waking on time;

8) sleep alone if possible;

9) keep your room temperature on the cool side. But sleep in bed socks if your feet get cold;

10) try adding copper and iron to your diet. A lack of them has been known to cause insomnia. Purchase them from your health store;

11) if you experience restless legs (a creepy-crawling sensation in your lower legs) ask your doctor to check for iron deficiency. It often causes such discomfort;

12) if you habitually waken after a couple of hours, get up, warm a cup of raw milk, add a teaspoon of raw honey,

take some deep breathing exercise, take a couple of herbal sleep tablets such as Good Nite, pray or meditate for a few minutes, then lie down and try sleep again;

13) try the homeopathic remedy called *Coffea*, under the tongue.

14) if you are subject to body aches, try an aspirin and a *DLPA* tablet at bedtime to quiet such pain, which could cause insomnia.

Snoring — If your own snoring wakes you, think what it must do to a sleeping partner. Or if your sleeping partner keeps you awake, try a new antisnoring medication called *Vocoslip*. It is a mixture that is placed in the nose before bedtime. It has proven effective for both men and women. Statistics show that everyone over 45, women included, snores, at least some of the time, because the mucous membranes in the nose and throat become dry during the night due to breathing through the mouth.

Not all people respond satisfactorily to Vocoslip, but the majority of those tested stopped their snoring. I have no knowledge of its ingredients, so be cautious. If they seem to be "natural," try it. There are also certain types of pillows now available which purport to stop snoring. I do not know their source, perhaps Swanson's Health Products.

Nervous Tension — Dr. Som was well aware — as are many other naturalists — that one of the causes of nervous tension is a spasm in the anus — the sphincter muscle. It is difficult to say which precedes the other, whether nervous tension causes the tightened muscle or vice versa. At any rate, they seem to go hand in hand. Dr. Som used to don a rubber glove and enter the tensed anus to massage gently on the inside. If the tension was so great that massage was impossible, he recommended the following:

Purchase a rectal dilator from the drug store. If one is

not available then use an ordinary enema tube, sold with douche bags. Lubricate it well with castor oil or wheat germ oil. Insert it carefully into the rectum and allow it to remain from 10 to 20 minutes. It should be inserted at least three inches. You may either lie on your left side or assume the knee-chest position. With the tube inserted about three inches it is coming in contact with an acupuncture point which relaxes the entire body so that nervous tension vanishes. Any time you feel "up-tight," unusually nervous, try this natural method, which should fully correct your problem.

A rectal tube sold as a device for healing hemorrhoids may be used for this purpose. It's called *Hemorr-ice*. For hemorrhoids it's supposed to be first placed in the freezer to cool the liquid sealed inside it. But cold isn't necessary for relaxing the sphincter muscle. If interested, the device may be ordered from Technology 2000 Corp. (Address elsewhere.)

Stress — Stress can be caused by subconsciously performed habits which tighten muscles and cause tension. Usually it is through a clenched jaw, which often becomes a habit rather than a reaction to tension and stress. First of all, learn to pause throughout the day to make sure you aren't clenching your jaw. The best way to achieve this is to put your lips lightly together while keeping the teeth slightly apart. Make sure the tongue gently touches the roof of the mouth just behind the top teeth. You'll find your jaw dropping comfortably. Just close your eyes and relax. If you will do this often for a week or so you'll find it becoming a habit which will greatly relieve stress and tension. It will also avoid problems with the teeth, which could become misaligned through jaw tension.

Fatigue and the Adrenal Glands — Fatigue is the name given to the ailment that descends upon us in a strange unexplainable manner. Unexplainable because the physician pronounces nothing drastically wrong, just a "need for rest." But very few physicians can point to the actual cause: a slowdown of the adrenal glands because they cannot operate at peak efficiency; they cannot continue to distribute the output of their priceless hormone — cortisone. Why? Because their natural functioning has been damaged by too many unnatural foods and drinks. Without the outflow of cortisone the body simply goes into a state of fatigue and depression. Your physician is right, you do need rest, but you certainly need a lot of other things. May I suggest methods of restoration.

1) During those days or weeks that you are resting and recuperating, avoid meat as much as possible and eat fruits, vegetables, grains, nuts, legumes with corn, raw cheese, tofu.

2) Add *pantothenic acid* and *vitamin* C to your diet; stimulants for the adrenal glands.

3) If your doctor agrees, also add *adrenal capsules*, available from your health store.

4) Order *Antifatigue* tablets from Hanna Kroeger. Or contact Michael Tierra for herbal therapies for stress, insomnia and fatigue. Also a natural stimulator for the adrenals.

5) *Damiana* capsules are excellent to restore nerve fatigue. They are available from your health store.

6) Your fatigue is no doubt also due to a lack of nerve vitality, meaning they have need of *lecithin*, which the body produces within itself. But because you have fed the body with too many processed foods and drinks it has ceased to produce its natural lecithin and the nerves thus cannot

project their nerve force. Lecithin will not only help restore the nerve energy but it acts as an emulsifying agent against a high cholesterol buildup in veins and arteries. Buy lecithin in micro-differential form from your health store, as granules. Take at least three teaspoons a day, swallowed with water, until your fatigue is healed. Then perhaps once a day.

7) To stimulate and restore adrenal action, begin a yogic asana (pose) called the *cobra pose* which requires very little energy but acts as a tremendous stimulant to the adrenals. I've just described how to perform it. (See Chapter 13 under *Sinus Congestion*.)

8) If you can bear the shock, finish your warm shower with a few seconds of a cold splash. The shock acts as a stimulant to the adrenals which will immediately begin to release an outflow of cortisone and, within a very few moments, you begin to feel an upsurge in energy and a sense of well-being.

9) Exercise. Walk, if possible, deep breathing occasionally. And, standing at an open window, simply take long, deep breaths, holding, and exhaling slowly. Or ride a bicycle, even a stationary kind.

Energy — When you need a quick energy pick up, reach for a piece of fruit with natural sugar instead of a bar of candy. Grapes in moderation are especially recommended, the grape sugar turning almost immediately into energy. Carrot juice is loaded with natural sugar. Bananas are excellent, containing not only a natural fruit sugar but calcium, potassium, phosphorus, vitamins A, B, C and iron. But be sure to eat only those bananas that are thoroughly ripened (turning brown), else they are still too acid. These fruits are the quick energy foods. If a bit of protein is desired with the fruit try a spoon of sesame-Tahini.

But for long-lasting energy try apples and raw natural cheese. And rely on starches — potatoes baked in the skin, whole grains, and root vegetables such as carrot, beet, parsnip, turnip, celery, jicama. The banana qualifies here, too. These are the foods that both heat the body and sustain energy — much to be desired over sugars because these starches require longer to digest, maintaining a natural level of blood sugar. They do not overtax the pancreas. Sixty-eight percent of all starches are converted into sugar. The thin outer coating of the skin of the potato should be removed by thoroughly scrubbing. Until then, the skin contains all manner of germs and pollutants. Eat the remaining surface skin. Actually the greatest source of the potato protein is found just beneath the skin, after the outer surface has been scrubbed away.

Preparing Rescue Remedy — Rescue Remedy is a famous homeopathic remedy that is taken in case of any injury and stress. It's a combination of: Clematic, Impatiens, Star of Bethlehem, Cherry Plum and Rock Rose. Purchase a bottle of Rescue stock, which will contain the five listed tinctures. Into a 1 ounce dropper bottle put 5 drops of Rescue stock. Fill the bottle with brandy or cider vinegar. Or, lacking the Rescue stock, into a 1 ounce dropper bottle, put 2 drops of each of the five ingredients, then fill with brandy or vinegar. Order from Standard Homeopathic (Hylande Brand) or Boericke & Tafel, Inc. (Alpha Brand). Or order Rescue Remedy already prepared from either of these companies.

For information concerning homeopathic products write to the Dr. Edward Bach Center or Herbal Home Products. Or for information concerning a homeopathic doctor write to the American Center for Homeopathy or the National Center for Homeopathy (addresses elsewhere).

Chapter Fifteen

Tooth and Gum Disease

A report by researchers at Indiana's Ball State University reveals that 50% of two year olds in America have cavities! And by the age of four 90% of all American children have dental decay! Less than 4% of our high school pupils are free of dental decay. Sixty percent of young adults, 80% of middle age adults and 90% of adults over age 65 have periodontal disease (pyorrhea), a gum disease. Doesn't speak well of our popular toothpastes and powders, does it? — those fluoride formulas — all that fluoridated water which was supposed to prevent or heal all our cavities!

The principal function of the teeth is to masticate our food. Thus, nature usually begins our life with good strong teeth. She first supplies the inner substance called dentine. Dentine is covered with a harder substance, enamel. Tooth enamel is the hardest substance found in the body. A tooth is composed of three portions: the root, which projects deep into the jawbone; the neck, which is that portion covered by the gums; and the crown. In spite of nature's efforts, the mouth is one of the most abused areas of our body. It is astonishing how nature protects us from our own foolishness. We place many wrong chemicals in the mouth. We drink liquids too hot or too cold. We brush with the wrong toothbrushes and we use the wrong toothpastes and powders.

We select a bad diet and the teeth respond since they are part of the whole person. Many diseases occur because of our diet and improper mouth habits. Millions lose their teeth, finding it necessary in order to restore health. They develop gum problems, cavities, pyorrhea and all manner of diseases. The gum tissues soften, allowing the teeth to drop.

The condition of the tongue reflects the condition in the stomach. Why do you suppose doctors frequently ask to see the tongue? They are observing its condition and are reading thereby the condition of the digestive system. If the tongue is coated, it indicates a problem in the stomach and intestines. A black tongue indicates problems in the lungs. Inflamed tissues indicate inflamed tissues in the stomach. Sores on the tongue indicate sores in the stomach. Minute ulcers on the tongue often indicate ulcers in the stomach, usually temporary.

Neglect of the teeth can cause decay, and decay will develop cavities. We look to our dentist to repair the damage but he can never correct the cause. Only you can do that. He can fill the cavity, to be sure, and attempt to heal the diseased gums. The cavity filling will only last a few years and must be repaired while the diseased gums may never be healed and you may lose your teeth. Assuredly, if you continue your bad eating habits, you will. One day the doctor will advise you that it is not wise to continue an attempt to save your teeth, it would be best to have them removed. Fortunately this happens less and less today since dentists know that extraction doesn't correct the cause of bad teeth.

In most cases it would be far better to keep them and attempt repair by a change to natural food and dental habits. Once the teeth are out the entire facial structure undergoes a change and there is often a perpetual struggle the rest of your life to obtain teeth that "fit."

Unless you have already had your teeth removed you may be able, through new dental technology, to save them throughout your lifetime. A tooth can now be saved even when the nerve is injured, either by deep decay or accidentally, even when the nerve becomes infected. Teeth should be extracted only under the most dire circumstances. Every effort should be made to save them since man has never successfully substituted false for the real product nature gave us.

Broken and diseased teeth and gums can often be cured by following a health routine — switching to a natural food diet, changing dental habits, exercise, and rest. Acupuncture treatments also are of tremendous value. Pause before removing even an abscessed tooth. First try a raw food diet and other dental steps before agreeing to removal. If there is healthy tissue remaining around the diseased tooth a good blood supply brought to it may eventually heal it. The teeth and gums themselves are seldom the direct cause of a disease or source of infection. They are only a repository where poisons that flow in the bloodstream collect. An abscess at the root of a tooth is a small ulcer. Why not attempt to cure it, rather than pull the tooth? Purify the bloodstream of toxins and there is every possibility the gums may be healed and all the teeth saved.

Restoring Health to Teeth and Gums

Today we hear that medical science has not yet discovered the cause of most dental problems, yet innumerable articles and books have been written focusing on a bad diet. The mystery is wondering why there is a mystery. Remembering that the teeth are a part of the whole person, since we are dealing with holistic or wholistic healing, we must consider the diet first. Teeth fed by a healthy bloodstream and thoroughly cleaned will never decay. Thus when attempting to heal periodontal disease the diet must be our first consideration.

It is redundant to dwell again on the three deadly whites and processed foods. Mention is made again only as a guideline toward a better diet. There are other significant points concerning the diet which have an impact upon healthy teeth. Periodontal disease is often related to osteoporosis. Very few doctors are aware that *the main cause of osteoporosis is excessive meat consumption.* Meat contains 22 times more phosphorus than calcium, creating an oversupply of phosphorus, which the human system cannot metabolize without a sufficient supply of calcium. The body, attempting to metabolize the excessive phosphorus, draws upon its own calcium reserves which creates severe calcium deficiencies in bone tissues, teeth and even hair. This leads eventually to periodontal disease and loss of teeth. And loss of hair. And osteoporosis.

Doctors usually respond by prescribing more and more calcium without ever once wondering what causes the deficiency in calcium. With the intake of calcium, arthritis often sets in — when actually the original cause is meat in the diet, meat with its oversupply of phosphorus and the body's attempt to balance it by drawing calcium from the bones. *The answer is not more calcium, but less meat.* One would do well to become a vegetarian but, failing that, to at least reduce meat consumption and concentrate more on seeds (such as sesame, sunflower and pumpkin), fruits, vegetables, nuts, tofu, meat substitutes, silica and magnesium supplements, raw milk and raw cheese, eggs and grains.

Vitamin supplements are an important part of a dietary program. When experiencing tooth decay consider adding vitamin B6 to the diet. When teeth become loose it indicates a lack of vitamin C. Bleeding gums may be aided by taking vitamin C with bioflavonoids included. A slow buildup of infection and inflammation, if not corrected, will cause loss of teeth. To overcome pyorrhea (periodontal disease) you need vitamin D in your diet. Good strong teeth require the presence of vitamin D. Expose the body, but not the face, to the sun early each day if possible or after 4:00 o'clock in the afternoon. Or take a vitamin D tablet.

Also, break open a vitamin E gelatin capsule and massage your gums with the oil. Or pop one in your mouth, break it open with your teeth and, with your tongue, spread the oil around your teeth and gums before swallowing the capsule. Or buy a bottle of vitamin E oil from your health store and massage your gums with it. With a corrected diet this could lead to the disappearance of gum problems.

As for cleaning the teeth, may I recommend a homemade formula for tooth powder which I concocted myself. I mix equal portions of Real Salt or Dews Salt with baking soda, myrrh and oak bark powder. To order Real Salt or Dews Salt, seek address elsewhere — or buy sea salt or any good mineral salt at your health store. The myrrh and oak bark powder can also be purchased at your health store.

Often oak bark isn't available in powder form, in which case buy the capsules and break them open. Mix the formula thoroughly. To destroy bacteria on your toothbrush dip it into a cup containing 3% hydrogen peroxide from the drug store, then dip your dampened toothbrush into the loose powder mixture. This homemade dentifrice has been known to cure many mouth problems. The ingredients of the powder are abrasive enough to remove any bacteria and actually kill it. The hydrogen peroxide releases oxygen bubbles that destroy bacteria.

About salt — when a doctor tells you to give up salt he or she means white refined table salt — or even sea salt. But there's a mineral salt, an alternative. Mineral salt is mined from rock salt that has all the natural minerals left in — the manganese, iron, magnesium, zinc, sulfur, copper, calcium, phosphorus, iodine. Ordinary refined white table salt is rock salt with all the other vital minerals "refined" out of it. *This* salt is dangerous. But the rock salt containing all the other minerals is a "good guy." Real Salt is such a product. Your health store probably sells Real Salt. If not, write to American Orsa, Inc., for a distributor in your area. Or you may prefer to order Mineral Salt from the Dews Company. (Addresses elsewhere.) Dews also sells an unrefined "white" sugar derived from vegetables.

When I was a child growing up at home, Mama mixed salt and soda with charcoal for our dentifrice. I don't know where she got the idea and I don't know where she got the charcoal. But if you'd like to try it, purchase charcoal capsules from the health store, break them open and mix the charcoal powder with salt and soda. Since then I've learned that charcoal whitens the teeth and kills impurities. Well, charcoal is often used to remove the impurities in water purifiers, so why wouldn't it also kill impurities in the mouth? Dip your dampened brush into salt-soda-charcoal as described above and brush after each meal, as you would with any other tooth powder.

If you're not "into" mixing formulas at home, then consider *Mer-flu-an*, a natural tooth powder. It's made of baking soda, sea salt, myrrh and peppermint. Not too different from my homemade formula. It's supposed to eliminate the hypersensitivity around exposed necks of teeth, and fight diseases of the periodontium (the tooth-holding structure). Available at your health store or from Swanson Health Products. (Address elsewhere.) Or purchase *Peelu* dentifrice from your health store. It's available in paste, powder, or liquid and it's excellent.

Without a doubt you already brush your teeth immediately upon arising. It's advisable to massage the gums at least once a day. Edgar Cayce recommended a product called *Perident* for massaging gums and destroying germs and bacteria responsible for gum disease. Order from wherever Cayce products are sold or from Cayce Corner in Phoenix. (Address elsewhere) Lacking Perident, you may want to try the following: After brushing, moisten a small portion of a washcloth with clear water and, with one finger, massage the gums up and away from the teeth. Also rub the teeth downward away from the gums. Massage vigorously.

The gums may bleed at first, but give it no thought. The massage is stimulating and increasing circulation. Projecting the tongue scrub the top of it vigorously with a fresh portion of the washcloth. Clean it thoroughly as far back as possible. This stimulation and removal of all the mucus from your mouth strengthens the muscles of your face, your mouth, your tongue, and your throat. It also helps prevent germs from finding a breeding ground for disease in the throat and mouth.

Now extend the tongue as far as possible, then, with muscles still tensed, raise the tip to the roof of the mouth as far back as possible. Continue this movement several times. This action is very good for the muscles of the throat and face, bringing youthful regeneration. Turn the tip of the tongue upward and rub the tip vigorously against the roof of the mouth, backward and forward. This action will stimulate an increased flow of saliva, which should be swallowed. Saliva thus created greatly increases digestion. Now grasp the tongue with the washcloth and pull outward with a stretching movement.

Again, secure a nasal douche or *Neti Pot* and flush the nasal passages with warm water with salt. I've described its use earlier in Chapter 13. This not only removes considerable mucus but also toxic acids that have settled in the nasal and sinus passages. (Never swallow loosened mucus.) You may never suffer sinus problems again, and it may be the procedure which will save your teeth. Now drink a couple of glasses of distilled water at room temperature. (Avoid tap water, if possible.)

Bad Breath — Halitosis means bad breath, something hardly anyone speaks about. Bad breath is caused by the growth of bacteria in your mouth. Bacteria needs to be broken up and rinsed away daily. It can certainly be destroyed by using the homemade formula I've suggested.

To fight bad breath a new electronic odor meter called *Doctor Ettequette* can quickly reveal the unpleasant truth. It's a device featuring a row of four colored lamps. When you exhale upon them they light up. Green 2 indicates zero odor. Green 1 means very slight. Yellow warns you need to rinse with a mouthwash. Red means... get lost.

The device resembles a tiny tape recorder. It's manufactured in Japan and should sell for about one hundred dollars. If you continuously come up red, you'd better see your dentist. Continued bad breath means your mouth needs immediate dental attention. Something is wrong. There could be embedded bacteria in your gums which could become a serious problem.

Bleeding Gums — Wash six lemons thoroughly in vinegar water, Clorox water or Amway's LOC to remove poisonous sprays. Then cut the lemons in small pieces. Place them in 1-1/2 quarts water and bring to a boil, remove from the heat and steep for 25 minutes, strain and allow it to cool. Drink 6 ozs. twice daily for ten days. If the gums are bleeding badly, apply the concoction to the gums with a cotton pat. The strong juice will do much to remove pus and congestion in the gums. Or, to repeat, massage with pure vitamin E oil, available from your health store. Or rinse your mouth with warm salt water four times a day. Or add salt to warm water in your Water Pik twice a day.

Broken Tooth — Save the tooth, rinse it with water or hydrogen peroxide, wrap it in a facial tissue and replace it in your mouth to keep it moist — then get to your dentist fast. It may be possible to implant your own tooth if you act quickly.

The Lemon Treatment — Dr. Som, always thinking first of natural remedies, found lemons to be effective in healing gum problems. Take pure lemon juice into the mouth, and hold it awhile, both morning and evening. It will reduce swelling and inflammation and drive the poisons back into the bloodstream where they can be expelled. With the mouth full of lemon juice, rinse the whole wall cavity with it. Be sure to rinse the mouth thoroughly immediately after discarding so that the lemon acids do no damage to the tooth enamel, preferably using water containing baking soda to neutralize the citric acid. Or use thick Milk of Magnesia to rinse the mouth after the lemon, but do not swallow the MOM because it contains aluminum. The acid of lemon and other citrus fruit is strong enough to affect tooth enamel.

After drinking a glass of orange juice, for instance, rinse the juice out thoroughly before brushing your teeth. If you do not you will be brushing much of the citrus acid into the enamel. After rinsing, you may choose to brush lightly with baking soda or my special homemade formula which contains soda, to destroy the acid. *Never, never leave citrus acid too long in the mouth, else it will "pit" your tooth enamel.* But used as a rinse as I have suggested, lemon juice is a deadly enemy to pus and phlegm. Lemon juice has been known to cure pyorrhea. The lemon juice will remove inflammation from around the gums and firm up flabby gum tissues.

Apply small strips of lemon to the gums and teeth and, with your finger, use it as you would a toothbrush, massaging and cleaning. You may place a slice of lemon over an infected tooth and leave it there a few minutes until the juice is all extracted. Several hours later, repeat this poultice treatment. Repeat it until the swelling is removed. Again, neutralize the citrus acids immediately with rinsing then brushing with baking soda.

Tartar deposits accumulate on teeth when the diet is wrong. There is too much uric acid. Again, meat is the culprit. Meat is filled with uric acid. Cleaning the teeth with lemons as you would a brush will usually remove tartar deposits. Again, rinse well and brush with baking soda to neutralize the acid.

Sensitive Teeth — Sensitive teeth are usually caused by overexposed roots and can be corrected. Such sensitivity means hot or cold substances can't be tolerated. They cause intense discomfort, even pain. A new dental treatment requiring only ten minutes helps six out of ten patients. The dentist applies a substance called *dipotassium oxalate* and allows it to soak into the teeth to create tiny crystals which form a protective barrier. Two minutes later a second coat is applied. This seals the teeth against exposure. Usually one such treatment suffices.

Sugarless Gum — Researchers state that chewing sugarless gum when you can't brush after a meal or snack will prevent cavities. Or chew a gum sweetened with *Xylitol*, a natural substance found in fruits and vegetables. It loosens plaque, making it easier to remove while brushing. I hesitate even to mention it since chewing gum is such a gross habit. If you do as suggested, please discard the gum soon. And don't chew gum in public. Did you ever notice that when an uncouth or unsavory character is portrayed in the movies, he or she is usually depicted chewing gum?

Chew a carrot or apple if possible, rather than gum. Many raw fruits and vegetables are natural teeth cleaners so bite directly into them rather than using a knife. If nothing is available, just rinse your mouth with water several times. It disturbs the bacteria buildup.

Tea Tree Oil — For mouth ulcers, sore gums, bad breath and plaque, dab Tea Tree Oil on the gums. If too strong dilute with water or vitamin E oil. Or add three drops to water and use as a mouthwash twice daily. See Chapter 18 for additional information on Tea Tree Oil.

Daily use of a *Water Pik* is a must, at least once a day. If you wish, add salt to the warm water — Epsom salt if you have high blood pressure. Use the Water Pik immediately after eating. The water wash will forcefully remove many particles the toothbrush cannot reach. It also stimulates the tissues and gums for better circulation. Then use a good mouthwash such as Plax or Listerine for loosening plaque, then brush your teeth. Or use *Glyco-thymoline*, available where Edgar Cayce products are sold, or, again, from Cayce Corner. But *do* use a good one constantly. Brush or floss immediately after using the mouthwash so that loosened plaque and bacteria may be brushed or flossed away.

Teething Pains — use a cold teething ring for teething infants. The cold helps the tender gums. Refrigerate the teething ring to keep it cold. Massage gums with warm castor oil, not enough oil to cause gagging.

Toothache — An ice cube again to the rescue! But, surprise, you don't apply it to your tooth. Instead you rub it for several minutes on the web of skin between the thumb and index finger of your hand — the one on the same side as your toothache. Other suggestions: cover tooth with a wad of pure cotton soaked in oil of cloves. Rinse with a solution of half and half warm water and hydrogen peroxide. Or place a piece of garlic in the cavity. Or boil a raisin or fig in milk and apply while hot.

Toothbrushes — Buy a new toothbrush every two weeks. Or soak your old one in powerful hydrogen peroxide to destroy bacteria and germs. Toothbrushes are breeding grounds for bacteria which create a chronic sore throat or gum infection. A good choice is a curried-bristle brush known as the *Collis-Curve* brush. It has a row of straight bristles in the center surrounded by rows of outside bristles curved inward. If unavailable at your stores, order from George Collis. (Address elsewhere.) Research has found this toothbrush to be far superior to others in removing plaque. You should have about four of these toothbrushes, used in rotation, giving each one an opportunity to dry thoroughly.

Natural bristles are usually not the best choice. They encourage the greatest growth of bacteria because they remain damp longer. The hollow core in each bristle draws water and holds it. Always choose soft bristles because they get at hard to reach areas and destroy colonies of bacteria and plaque.

When brushing, avoid sawing back and forth. Rather, rotate the motion almost up and down. This will not only remove food particles but will also massage the gums. It's called "sulcus" brushing. Insert the bristles at a 45 degree angle and wiggle the bristles as if to dislodge plaque and food housed between the teeth or along the gum line and to attack bacterial colonies nesting around the stem of the teeth. A series of such wiggles should be effective, moving from one tooth to the next. Form a habit of sulcus brushing. Keep a toothbrush at your place of employment. Frequently dip the brush in a sterilizer, such as hydrogen peroxide, to kill bacteria. Or place the toothbrush in a container of hydrogen peroxide after each brushing for constant sterilization. Thus you don't have to buy new toothbrushes so often.

Try to brush after each meal. Not only should you have a toothbrush at your site of employment as well as at home, but you should keep extra floss at both places. Floss at least once a day, because bacterial colonies form rapidly on the teeth and must be removed daily. Use unwaxed floss. Always floss at bedtime.

There is now a product called *Super Floss* you may want to try, especially if you have bridges. Or use *Stimudent*.

If your gums continue to bleed and evidence inflammation, see your doctor for a blood, urine, saliva and hair analysis. Check for vitamin, mineral, enzyme and glandular deficiencies.

Root Canals

Most controversial! Many dentists perform a root canal without a second thought — and many root canals are successful. But many are not. Why? Because the infection at the root of the tooth remains undetected even though the dentist sincerely tries to remove all of it. After sealing the dead tooth, the infection seeps into the jaw bone and into the bloodstream.

If you suspect this is happening your dentist can perform an apicoectomy which removes the infected root tip and the cyst, often saving the tooth. But more often, health problems develop throughout the body without the least suspicion that the dead tooth and its infected root could be at fault. Acupuncture meridians run throughout the body linking every tooth with various organs. So organs far removed from the infected tooth could be affected. For instance, kidney problems could be related to an infected root canal.

Electroacupuncture has fairly recently appeared on the dental scene to aid in detecting the problem. It's done through the use of a Voll machine which measures the energy level of a tooth to determine if it is acting as a focus of infection and creating problems in distant parts of the body. If it proves to be the culprit, you have two choices.

One, you can have the dead tooth removed, making very sure the infected bone around the tooth is also removed, else it will continue to spread low-grade infection to distant parts of the body.

Or, two, you can ask for a homeopathic remedy to hopefully heal the infected root. If it fails to do so the tooth must be pulled. I have said elsewhere never to pull a tooth if it can be saved, but it may be better to lose an infected dead tooth than to have a low-grade infection leaking constantly into the body, creating hard-to-diagnose problems. There is every hope the homeopathic remedy can heal the infection.

"Silver" Fillings

Fillings in the teeth should contain no "silver" or amalgam. Silver is a definite poison — because it's not really silver, it's mercury. The student dentist is told never to handle scrap amalgam — the part left over after filling a tooth with silver. Gloves must be worn while handling, then it must be stored under water in a sealed container until the health department of your community can pick it up for recycling. This dread mercury material must never be touched or left in an open container or thrown in the trash. Yet this deadly amalgam has just been used to fill a tooth.

The American Dental Association assures both the dentist and the patient that the deadly mercury in the patient's mouth is securely sealed in the hardened filling and is therefore safe for the patient. But is it? "They" say research has proved mercury to be undetectable after amalgam hardens. But other research has also proven that the mercury can "leak" and unbound mercury is one of the most deadly of our poisons. One half the amalgam in a silver tooth filling is mercury.

Shortly after mercury was introduced into dentistry,

in the early 1800s, the first case of multiple sclerosis was documented. Currently, those dentists who are removing "silver" fillings from their patients' mouths are finding that all manner of "incurable" diseases suddenly go into remission. Anyone experiencing a "mystery" illness, one for which the doctor can find no obvious cause, should look to his or her teeth. The mercury in their amalgam fillings may be leaking into the bloodstream. Should a doctor tell you the disease you have has no known cure — that you'll just have to live with it — look to your teeth.

Do be aware that there is a wrong and right way to remove silver fillings and not all dentists are qualified to remove them. Seek one who knows the proper procedure. And one who is aware that with the removal of such a filling, the patient could suffer a reaction for a few days due to the exposure of the dangerous metal during removal. You should prepare beforehand with massive doses of vitamin C and minerals. Be prepared to take a colonic to eliminate the poisons should one be indicated. If the proper procedure for removing silver fillings is not followed you could suffer from even worse symptoms.

Your selected dentist would have in his office or could direct you to a dentist with an instrument called an *amalgameter.* With this device, he measures the electrical current of each metal filling. The current output, ranging from 0 to 50 microamperes, could be either positive or negative. The filling registering the highest negative reading must be removed first. Next, the one registering the next highest negative, until all the negatives have been removed, ending with the filling registering the lowest negative. Only then should the positive fillings be removed, beginning with the highest positive and removing last the filling with the lowest positive.

During the removal process continue massive intake of vitamin C and minerals. After each removal take homeopathic *Merc Salve* to overcome the effects of any mercury in your system.

Once a filling is removed it should be replaced with either gold or composite (a mixture of a quartz ceramic and an epoxy acrylic resin) or porcelain fused to gold, or a ceramic called Cerestore. Reject nickel, it's almost as bad as silver. Ask for a filling with NO metals. Dicar, a porcelain-like material, is often used. If using gold, always use gold without palladium. Gold with palladium collects currents. Add porcelain if you wish, but never aluminum. Reject all metals. They aren't necessary.

Diseases known to improve or disappear after the removal of silver fillings are: multiple sclerosis, leukemia, numbness of hands and feet, neurological problems, tremors, speech disorders, mental and emotional disorders such as depression, anxiety, suicidal tendencies, immune system malfunction lowering the body's ability to resist disease, cardiovascular problems, inability to walk (Parkinson's disease?), epilepsy, loss of memory and other mental problems such as confusion, irritability and depression. (Alzheimer's?)

Don't be afraid to tell your dentist not to use silver amalgams in your filling. If he insists on doing so seek another dentist. There are enough holistic dentists now available so that we no longer have to tolerate those who "have eyes but refuse to see." And the next time you need an old filling replaced make very sure it's replaced with a nonmetallic material or with gold. For more information about "silver" fillings, do read *It's All In Your Head*, a book by Dr. Hal Huggins, a recognized leader in the battle against mercury. His address is in the last chapter.

For the name of a holistic dentist in your area, call Dr. Joel Berger of Bayside, NY; Dr. Michael Ziff of Orlando, FL; or Dr. Mark Hulet of Victorville, CA. Their phone numbers can be found in the last chapter. I know Dr. Hulet personally. He is very knowledgeable concerning holistic dentistry.

TMJ

It's unbelievable how many people suffer from imbalance of the temporomandibular joint — or TMJ — without even knowing it. This joint is located just in front of each ear where the lower jaw is hinged to the skull. The effects of a malfunctioning TMJ joint projects through the whole system, causing distress throughout the body. If you suffer from any of the following, see your dentist and ask to be referred to a TMJ specialist:

1) Headaches — especially migraines or any one-sided headache. Stress can follow a TMJ dysfunction, causing pain in all muscles of the head, ear, neck and shoulder. It can cause misalignment of the teeth. A good TMJ specialist can fit you with a splint which, worn in the mouth over the teeth for several months, can adjust and correct the problem. It may be necessary to have your teeth crowned to hold them in alignment.
2) Tense jaw muscles.
3) Grinding or gnashing the teeth.
4) Loss of hearing.
5) Difficulty in opening your mouth due to a painful jaw.
6) A crooked smile.
7) One eyebrow lower than the other.

TMJ can cause neck and facial pains which can be misdiagnosed as arthritis. It can cause unrelated earaches, sinus pain and inability to close the mouth, headaches that resemble migraine, facial pain mimicking a tic douloureux, or temporal arthritis, neck and shoulder pain, dizziness, tinnitus (ringing in the ear), subjective hearing loss. TMJ can be caused from a blow to the head or jaw or from opening the jaw too wide or too long when biting or yawning. A maladjusted bite can cause trouble also. It frequently happens when a tooth is lost and not replaced, through moving the lower jaw out of position and misaligning the joint.

A common cause is clenching or gnashing the teeth when under tension or stress. The TMJ problem is finally beginning to be recognized. Although it may be difficult to find a knowledgeable dentist for relieving the pain, adjusting the bite and reestablishing joint alignment, TMJ specialists are becoming more numerous.

When all else fails there is now offered to patients a special type of artificial joint surgery. Experts can now replace deteriorated jaw joints with new artificial ones that relieve the dreadful pain of TMJ. The artificial joint is implanted through tiny incisions at the base of the jaw and in front of the ear. It is held in place by small screws. Eventually the body's own tissue grows into the joint's porous ends, forming a tight permanent bond. It requires only two or three days hospitalization. If you are interested in further information concerning this procedure either you or your doctor should contact the TMJ Foundation, address in last chapter. Also ask your dentist about a new device called an *arthrophonometer*, which provides an accurate diagnosis of TMJ.

Dental Updates

Bedtime Bottles — Don't give junior or junioress a bottle of sweetened formula at bedtime. Continually sucking on it can develop jaw problems, and perpetual contact with sweets could cause early cavities. Results: destroyed baby teeth and misalignment of a jaw bone which could disfigure the child's face and affect the placement of incoming permanent teeth. Daytime formulas are no threat to teeth because saliva neutralizes the liquid. Not so at night. Give instead a pacifier. Breast-fed babies have straighter teeth because of more vigorous sucking, which develops stronger mouth and jaw muscles and promotes tooth alignment. Bottle-fed babies often have crooked teeth.

Decay Removed Without Drilling — An amazing new substance has been discovered which removes decay without drilling. It's called *GK-101E*. It actually attacks decay inside the tooth and carries it away, without harming healthy tissue. It's totally safe. It's been successfully tested in Japan and is now being tested here. Watch for its release to patients very soon.

Detecting Gum Disease — A hand held electronic device slightly larger than a fountain pen is enabling dentists to discover gum disease and treat it long before it becomes serious. It's called the *Periotest*. As the dentist taps each tooth with it a synthetic voice announces numbers that indicate how firmly the tooth is anchored to the jawbone. It's far superior to the X-ray, which only detects loose teeth when they are obvious.

Electronic Dental Anesthesia — is a new procedure that by-passes needles and numbness. A sticky pad is attached to the gums. It delivers a low-level electronic current that kills pain. If pain begins, the voltage is simply increased. Novocain is unnecessary.

Kissing — can transmit bacteria from one person to another. Saliva can contain millions of bacteria. So be sure your partner is fastidious about his/her mouth. The question of whether or not AIDS can be transmitted through kissing has never been satisfactorily answered. It's fairly certain that saliva is not a carrier. But what about rare mouth ulcers or wounds that tend to bleed? Just a thought.

Marijuana — People who smoke marijuana have been shown to have a greater number of filled teeth, decayed and missing teeth and more severe cases of gum disease. Marijuana apparently causes a greater accumulation of plaque and inflammation of the gums if smoked frequently.

Miracle Mouthwash — includes nothing more than a gargle with salt water. The solution is then studied by a computer which is able to detect diseases, such as hemophilia and sickle cell anemia.

This "miracle mouthwash" also has many other uses around the house — bleeding gums, colds, sore throats, congestion, and bad breath. But be careful not to swallow any of the salt water as it can be harmful to anyone with certain medical conditions. A saline solution can also be used to reduce bleeding and infections.

Oral Cancer — Vitamin E has been known to prevent cancer of the mouth. Tests given to hamsters proved that it helps to prevent the formation of mouth cancer. Two groups of hamsters were given a substance known to cause mouth cancer. One group, however, was also given vitamin E supplements. This group showed no indication of tumor formation after 22 weeks into the experiment. The other group developed one or more. The medical profession also believes vitamin E may help to prevent cancer elsewhere in the body. The usual dosage is 400 IUs a day. To repeat, massage gums with vitamin E oil — it could perhaps prevent or heal mouth cancer

Pain Killer — The needle which kills the pain is almost as bad as the pain it kills. Available is a new anesthesia which requires a fine, short needle to painlessly inject enough Novocain to numb only an area around a single tooth, eliminating numbness of lips, tongue and cheek. A new cherry-flavored mouthwash deadens the gums so that even the thin needle doesn't hurt. If there's swelling apply cold compresses to the outside of your cheek instead of placing aspirin on gums or aching tooth. Alternating hot and cold applications could do much to relieve pain.

Tooth Decay — A new antiseptic varnish called *Chlorzoin* is now being used to paint the teeth to prevent cavities. It slowly releases a germ killer on and into the teeth, destroying bacteria which causes decay. Its use can save pain and heavy dental expense in cavities, root canals, crowns, caps or false teeth, according to Canadian researchers.

Precautions in Dentistry

According to Dr. Donald Morse, professor of endodontology at Temple University, Dr. Anthony Di Angelis, associate professor of dentistry of the University of Minnesota, and Dr. Ronald Mitsuyasu, assistant professor of medicine at UCLA, dentists can certainly transmit all manner of disease to you and vice versa unless precautionary measures are taken. These diseases include: herpes, tuberculosis, mononucleosis, influenza, hepatitis, measles, syphilis, gonorrhea and AIDS. The precautionary measures include:

a) wearing rubber gloves by all dental staff members when working on patients;
b) wearing surgical masks while working on patients;
c) using disposable needles;
d) vaccination of the entire dental team against hepatitis B, the viral disease most commonly passed between dentist and patient.

Since blood is frequently drawn during a dental procedure, it would seem absolutely essential that the dentist wear gloves during any such procedure.

Chapter Sixteen

Common Infections

Candida Albicans (Yeast Fungus) — is a single cell fungus. They live inside the body and on the skin from the moment of our birth. In healthy individuals with strong immune systems they dwell within us and on the skin quite normally. But when the immune system weakens, when the natural balance of the body is disturbed, when the glands no longer distribute the proper hormones, the fungus multiplies rapidly. It first attacks the mucous membranes, and if not brought under control, can take over control of the entire body in only a few months.

The immune system includes clusters of cells and molecules throughout the body and white blood cells. The immune system's principal function is to differentiate between normal cells and foreign substances that invade the body and to destroy the invading substances.

There are several causes for a weakened immune system. One is improper nutrition — that is, fast foods, processed foods, polluted foods. Second is the intake of drugs administered by the conventional doctor, such as antibiotics, cortisone, and steroids. Birth control pills can also negatively affect the immune system. Stress in our day-to-day life style can also trigger destructive patterns. Diabetics are subject to candida. The candida itself can be a toxin.

About antibiotics — fungus infections very often follow after a doctor has given antibiotics, sulfa drugs, penicillin, or any of the so-called wonder drugs. These drugs may be effective in destroying whatever the problem was, but they also destroy the "good" lactic acid bacilli in the intestinal tract. This intestinal flora is a protection against infection and if the good flora has been destroyed the fungus flourishes. Therefore, immediately upon beginning or following any form of antibiotics, be very sure to take acidophilus capsules. Holistic physicians are very aware of this need but the usual allopathic physician often is not.

Since you must bring the candida under control, and since you must build up your immune system, may I suggest several methods of overcoming your problem:

1) You may wish to see your doctor if you have a vaginal or jock itch. The male's yeast infection is easily observable and treated. Not so, the female. The doctor must take substance from the vagina for a test similar to a pap smear. If the diagnosis is positive the doctor will prescribe a drug, often *Nystatin*. He may give you Nystatin tablets for oral medication plus Nystatin vaginal suppositories for killing the infection in the vagina. Nystatin works very slowly and often requires several months to establish a healing. Even then the infection often recurs. Some doctors prescribe a product called *Candex*, along with Nystatin capsules.

2) Candida calls for a change in your diet. Since yeast grows readily on simple sugar, avoid the simple sugar foods

in the diet which are: fruits, cakes, sweet rolls, candy, dairy products containing sugar, such as ice cream and sweetened yogurt, sugar in coffee. Your doctor may ask you to forego all dairy products. Also foods containing yeast, such as breads, alcoholic beverages, aged cheese and spaghetti. Avoid chocolate like the plague. Avoid wheat products and grains, fruit juices and nuts.

3) Purchase odor-free garlic capsules (health store).

4) Begin drinking Taheebo tea (*Pau d'arc*)

5) Build up your immune system. Write Hanna Kroeger (address elsewhere) and explain your problem to her. She will forward herbal products and homeopathic remedies that will destroy the fungus and build up your immune system. Her herbal products are *Kantita* and *Foon Goos*, which quickly detoxify the system and then destroy the fungus. Plus she will provide you with her special acidophilus tablet which you should take continuously to make sure the fungus does not return. It's called *Taurindophilus*.

6) Inquire concerning a tablet called *PM-7*, which is a drug to heal the infection. Its main ingredient is *Candicidin*, which is a heptaene macrolide naturally produced by fermentation. It is obtainable by writing: Health Information Service. (Address elsewhere.)

7) Next, you may wish to take *Echinacea* herb tablets which combat the growth of bacteria and fungus. It is excellent in building the immune system.

8) Since candidiasis fungus can be present throughout the body without obvious symptoms, common signals to observe are chronic heartburn, gastritis, colitis, gas, constipation, diarrhea, headaches, depression, hyper-irritability, memory loss, inability to concentrate, hay fever, sinusitis, earaches, hives, asthma, sensitivity to certain

foods and chemicals, yeast vaginitis, menstrual irregularities, cramping, endometriosis, cystitis, kidney and bladder infections, fatigue, joint pains and stiffness, cold hands and feet, increased body hair, numbness and tingling, food cravings, loss of libido.

9) Avoid all antibiotics, such as penicillin, ampicillin, tetracycline, erythromycin, amoxicillin and keflex. Also avoid immuno-suppressants such as cortisone, prednisone, and other steroid type medications. Avoid the birth control pill which contributes to candidiosis by upsetting the hormone balance.

10) Do ask your doctor to place you on an individualized program of vitamins, minerals, food concentrates, digestive enzymes and raw glandulars; based on your symptoms, hair analysis, blood and urine samples and genetic strengths and weaknesses determined by body measurements.

11) Take additional vitamin C, silica and magnesium. Also vitamin A and B complex. Fanie offers an excellent vitamin B complex in tincture form to be dropped under the tongue.

12) Avoid all forms of zinc since zinc has been known to promote the growth of candida.

13) *Caprylic acid*, also called octanoic or octylic acid, can be a major part of preventing the return of candida. It has the ability to slow the yeast's reproduction and destroy adult yeast cells. Sodium caprilate is also effective against Thrush, a candida infection of the throat, mouth and digestive tract. It can also be applied topically to fungal infections of the skin, such as athlete's foot and jock itch.

14) You may wish to try *PAA*, a product available from Dynapro International (address elsewhere). Ask for information concerning their other excellent products.

The PAA formula is supposed to be effective in healing stubborn cases of yeast infection throughout the body. Whereas most approaches require several months of special dieting and careful medication, PAA is said to be effective within two weeks. Do ask for full information about the product before taking.

15) Do not wear nylon underpants or lycra blend sports tights. Choose cotton underwear instead.

16) Do not use perfumed or antibacterial douches. These products destroy natural protection. Yogurt douches are excellent. Yogurt contains lacto bacilli which destroys harmful bacteria. A yogurt douche consists of 8 ounces of plain, unflavored yogurt with just enough water added to make it a running fluid. The best plan is to insert the mixture into the vagina at bedtime, using a douche bag, since the longer it remains in the vagina, the better the results. Cover with a sanitary napkin and leave overnight.

The douche should be repeated twice a week until the problem is solved. If yogurt is unavailable, use plain water with one teaspoon of white vinegar to restore acidity in the vagina. Never use apple cider vinegar as a vaginal douche. It encourages the growth of fungus.

17) *Cranberry capsules* are useful since they contain a natural organic benzoate effective in healing infections. Cranberries also help to heal internal infections, ulcers, diverticulitis, bladder infections, bleeding of the gums.

18) *Hydrogen peroxide* is very effective for healing yeast infection and restoring the immune system. Never take over-the-counter hydrogen peroxide. It's not meant for internal use. You must take a "food grade" peroxide. It can now be taken in subtle forms not offensive to the taste, such as *Stabilized Oxygen*. The usual dosage is ten drops in water twice a day, but an increased dosage may be

necessary for a few days to combat the yeast. Consult the firm from which you order it. You can also make a douche with one teaspoon of Stabilized Oxygen, three tablespoons of Aloe Vera gel or juice, and a half cup of water. Insert it into the vagina with a baby syringe. Stabilized Oxygen is available from Aerobic Life Products, Inc. (Address elsewhere)

19) The Women's Health Institute offers two products to overcome yeast infection: *Yeast Gard* and *Dual Gard*. Yeast Gard is a pure homeopathic formula in suppository form. Its purpose is to treat vaginal infections caused by candida. Dual Gard is a two capsule formula consisting of triglandular amino acids, minerals, and cell salts, formulated in a base of barley green, alfalfa and buckwheat. Both of these compounds may be ordered through Swanson's. (Address elsewhere.)

20) A new drug called *Terazol 7* is proving effective in the treatment of yeast infections. Another is *Terconazole*.

21) Avoid the use of tampons while under treatment.

22) Avoid sexual intercourse.

23) Cleanse the vulva and anal area after each bowel movement.

The female is called upon to endure yeast infections, so common in the female and considerably more rare in the male, simply because she has a vagina. Irritation and inflammation of the vagina and the flare-up of yeast infection is becoming increasingly common. Symptoms may be recognized by a vaginal discharge, itching, soreness and a burning sensation when urinating. These same symptoms can be caused by any number of other problems. A simple pap type test can quickly determine whether or not the problem is yeast infection.

Another vaginal problem is trichomoniasis, which is

almost always sexually transmitted — in which case the woman gets one infection after another, unwittingly transmitted by her sexual partner, who himself has trichomoniasis, although there is no evidence of a problem. *Metronidazole* is a drug given orally as an effective medication against trichomoniasis. The male sex partner should certainly also take the medication to prevent transmitting recurring infections to the female, who will also suffer bladder infections. Candidiosis, or yeast infection, usually evidences similar symptoms, so a doctor should never assume a vaginal problem to be caused by a bladder inflammation. *A bladder inflammation would be treated by an antibiotic, but a yeast infection would be made considerably worse. So a test similar to a pap smear could determine the answer.*

Again, the male partner should certainly submit to taking medication if the female experiences recurring candida or bladder infections. Although Nystatin cream applied topically will usually quickly heal the local problem in the male, he may have yeast infection throughout his body and be totally unaware. Diagnosing it is extremely difficult, but if he is experiencing fatigue or other symptoms with no apparent cause, and if his female partner is experiencing recurring candida (yeast) or bladder infections, he should take medication to destroy the fungus rampant through his immune system.

Nystatin suppositories are often used in combating candidial infections, but the FDA has approved other antifungal medications such as *Miconazole* or *Clotrimazole* and creams applied topically to the vulva or in vaginal suppositories. One single 500 milligram tablet of Clotrimazole has been found to be as effective in curing the infection as long term therapy. A drug called *Terconazole* seems to have replaced Nystatin as the best prescription drug presently to heal yeast infections.

Pelvic Infections — Women are particularly subject to pelvic infections. They include: vaginitis, pelvic inflammatory diseases and papillomavirus or genital warts. Vaginitis is usually caused by a flare-up of bacteria in the vagina. That's what vaginitis is: inflammation of the vagina. Again, it can be caused as a result of taking antibiotics which destroy good bacteria throughout the system.

Or it can be caused by a sexual partner who is infected and who unwittingly has deposited bacteria with his sperm into the female vagina. Or it can be because the immune system is so depleted the body itself cannot battle the inflammation. Or it can be caused by low estrogen levels. Or by allergies to vaginal sprays and deodorants.

Women have often been told that they can reduce pelvic inflammatory diseases and genital warts by avoiding sex with multiple partners but this is certainly not true. As stated above, her one male partner can carry in his own system for years a yeast or bacterial infection unknown to himself and to his female partner, or his semen may contain a "hidden" toxin that causes recurring bladder problems to the female. If a woman with only one sex partner experiences recurring pelvic problems she should insist that her male partner be thoroughly checked as a possible cause of her problems.

Warts in the Vagina — are due to viruses. Your doctor can treat them with *elector desiccation* under local anesthetic. But once they are removed they can recur. Do contact Hanna Kroeger or Michael Tierra to obtain advice concerning a method of destroying the viruses which cause the warts in the first place. Vaginismus, or painful intercourse is caused obviously by decreased vaginal secretions and changes in the lining of the vagina. It usually can be treated by inserting estrogen suppositories in the vagina.

Recently approved by the FDA are injections of *alpha interferon*, a protein that fights virus infections. The interferon is injected directly into the warts. This treatment is more effective than freezing, burning or chemical peel which have previously been used to prevent a recurrence of warts.

Fungus Infection (on the surface) — Some persons are more susceptible to fungus than others, and this susceptibility can be heightened by such conditions as heat and moisture. It most frequently occurs on the scalp, hands, feet or nails. The infection can be stubborn, and only in recent years has medication been developed which can control the more resistant cases. *Griesofulvin* has serious side effects. It is reputed to cause cancer. Avoid its use. You have other alternatives. A drug called *Naftin* is usually effective in treating athlete's foot, jock itch and other body fungus infestations. Fungus infection is contagious. Although the infection is rarely a life threatening health problem it should be treated by a doctor — not only because of its discomfort but because if it is not treated it might infect others.

Fungus infection of the scalp can be a very contagious disease in children. When a child is infected, patches of baldness may appear. These patches are round, gray and scaly, with a covering of tiny hairs which have been broken off at the scalp surface. The patches are about the size of a small coin bordered with tiny, itchy blisters. This type of infection usually appears on the face or neck, but it may occur on any part of the body. A scalp infection may spread from one child to another if they use each other's comb or brush, wear each other's hats or lean back against contaminated high-backed seats in classrooms, automobiles, theaters, etc. A child may get the infection from a cat, dog or other pet.

Sometimes it becomes "ringworm." Ringworm is a contagious fungus infection, a skin disorder which is misleadingly named. It is not caused by a worm, and the lesions are not necessarily ringed. It is quite common. Try castor oil applications. If not effective, see your doctor.

Tea Tree Oil — An effective product in combating internal or external fungus infections is *Tea Tree Oil*, which I have mentioned many times throughout this book. For external fungus infection of any kind, simply dab some on until the infection goes away. For minor vaginal infections, simply make a douche solution by adding five drops of the pure oil to 1/2 quart of water. Or add five drops to a sitz-bath. *Always* dilute the oil before using in the vagina. There will be a slight tingly feeling in the area. To obtain Tea Tree Oil or more information concerning it, see Chapter 18.

Chapter Seventeen

Healing Through Foods

The Fiber Foods — What about fiber foods, especially bran, about which there is such controversy?

Wheat grain is processed to two separate parts — the center, and the outer layer or germ. The center is ground to produce white flour. White flour contains a high degree of starch and very little real nutrients. It also contains a phosphorus compound which combines with important minerals — zinc, calcium, iron — and carries them out of the body with waste elimination, preventing their absorption in the bloodstream. Thus white bread and white flour pastries should be studiously avoided. Pure whole wheat, the outer layer or germ, contains the bran. Bran contains all of the essential B vitamins. It also contains protein, fat and vitamin E.

The mineral content in bran is equally impressive, namely phosphorus, potassium, iron and magnesium. Bran contains more of these minerals than any other food except yeast. The protein content is 16 grams to 1/2 cup. Fiber is absolutely essential for a healthy colon and intestinal tract — and bran is one of the prime sources of fiber food. The fiber content of bran prevents many digestive disorders and corrects some that are already in evidence. Some of these diseases are colitis, constipation, hernia, irritated bowel, spastic colon, diverticulitis, hemorrhoids, appendicitis, ulcers, varicose veins.

If you habitually eat whole grain bread, don't worry about the intake of bran, but usually only at a health store can such bread be obtained. Supermarket bread usually is "enriched" with the wrong substances, or it contains sugar and too much salt. If you consume a slice or so daily of whole grain bread that's all you need of fiber food. If not, perhaps you should add a spoon of bran regularly to some portion of your food. It is difficult to be specific as to the amount. It will depend upon the regularity of your particular elimination. If you are inclined to constipation, more may be necessary. If you are fairly regular, bran in moderation should be adequate. Within a few days, bowel action should become normal and diarrhea should disappear.

Be cautious of processed "all-bran" cereals, they may contain sugar. What you should search for is unprocessed bran and it usually is only available from your health store. If your doctor has placed you on a gluten-free diet you should avoid eating bran foods that contain gluten. Turn instead to brown rice, millet or corn meal cereals or bread. Or to the ground flaxseed that I spoke about at length in Chapter 4.

Bran may be added to casseroles, salad dressings, gravies, sauces, breads, cakes, meat loaves, omelets, scrambled eggs. If you eat cereal for breakfast mix in a spoon of bran. Add it to any beverage prepared in your blender or mix it with your milk or fruit juices once a day. The alarming decline of American health has sent researchers as far away as Africa attempting to discover whether or not diet is directly related to the problems of digestion. Africans, it was discovered, consume a lot of fibrous food. They have remarkably few cases of colon cancer, constipation, heart disease, appendicitis — while Westerners consume very little fiber and are beset not only with these diseases but many others.

Fibrous food is roughage. Fibrous food plays an important role in good health. It adds bulk to the diet. In the intestines fibrous food absorbs water and prevents constipation. Constipation leads to intra-abdominal pressure which pushes the stomach up through the diaphragm, resulting in hiatus hernia with its distressing heartburn, regurgitation of stomach acid, burning pain in back of the breast bone, dilated veins resulting in varicose veins and hemorrhoids.

When the colon is sluggish and food remains in the intestinal tract too long constipation is the result. Hard stools contain more bacteria and their sluggish movement through the intestines allows the bacteria to produce cancer-causing chemicals. Fibrous food changes all that. It causes the digestive juices to flow more vigorously, accelerates waste products through the system, and sweeps out encrusted waste products.

Research indicates the chances of heart attack are greatly reduced when one eats fibrous foods even in moderation. Fiber speeds the passage of food through the body. In addition to improving digestion the body does not absorb as many calories. One of the principal ways that fiber affects heart disease is by eliminating fats from the body.

Research also indicates that deaths from blood clots following surgery are reduced to zero if patients are put on a high fiber diet of whole wheat bread and bran. Blood clots which lodge in the lungs and the heart are the dominant cause of death following surgery. But a high fiber diet has proved amazingly successful in eliminating this hazard. During surgery the blood becomes more stagnant and apt to form clots because anesthetizing the patient causes total paralysis. Thus, during your recovery, there must be a good flow of blood through the veins.

A high fiber diet causes easy evacuation of the bowels, which is absolutely necessary because irregularity and constipation lead to blood clotting. Bran or flaxseed has been found to be much more successful than harsh laxatives which often lead to other problems. All this adds to its importance, not only following surgery but in daily use.

Having expressed praise concerning this wonderful food I must now add a word of caution. Some sensitive digestive systems find that bran foods produce gas, usually because they do not chew the foods long and well. Grain foods *must* be well salivated in the mouth before they enter the stomach area or problems could develop. The roughage could be too much for some rectal walls, creating problems in the rectum. So chew bran foods well. If problems develop with bran then choose flaxseed.

Much of the ordinary wheat germ sold on the market is made from wheat that is not organic; the wheat is fumigated and often sprayed before being made into wheat germ. A lot of the spray settles into the germ of the wheat. Bran may be an irritant to the stomach because of the dust and dirt left in it. So choose your brands carefully.

Wheat germ oils must also be used cautiously because of rancidity. Once the germ is separated from the wheat it is very subject to rancidity and rancid oils are a big factor in health problems. So be sure to purchase in small amounts, keep it refrigerated, and discard it should it not be used while still fresh. Bran can also be an irritant to the eyes if one is allergic to wheat. So before plunging into a bran/wheat germ program check as to allergies. And observe any "side effects." For the majority they are excellent foods. But for a few, as with all foods, they may be hazardous.

There are other fiber foods that work equally well if you cannot tolerate the brans, whole grain cereals and wheat germ. I've already mentioned prunes. Or concentrate on the flaxseed program previously mentioned. Or steel cut oatmeal from your health store. Excellent! Also try dates instead of jelly with your toast — or honey. Or jelly made with honey. Eat avocado often, too, which is an excellent natural laxative food. Eat ground peanuts occasionally for more roughage.

Fiber and Obesity — Too much food obviously contributes to obesity but the wrong kinds of food may be equally responsible. If the diet contains too little fibrous food, such as the proper kinds of grains, raw vegetable salads, potatoes, fruits, and too many refined foods which are depleted of fibers, such as pastries, sugars, and white flour, then the diet is contributing to obesity.

Fibrous foods produce four results.

1) They reduce the chances of overeating because they demand more chewing, thus slowing the intake.

2) They expand in your stomach to prevent overeating. Thus they are an excellent addition for a reducing diet.

3) They reduce the absorption of food from the intestinal tract.

4) They stimulate secretions that distend the stomach and induce a feeling of fullness. Research assuredly has proven that those whose diet includes refined foods soon

become hungry again and eat more often. When vegetables or grains are eaten one does not soon become hungry again.

Doctors invariably place their obese patients on diets with restricted carbohydrates yet in primitive societies, where obesity is rare, large quantities of carbohydrates are consumed. The difference is that their carbohydrates have built-in fibers — their grain cereals have not been refined and they eat many raw vegetables. The bulk factor in their diet prevents them from overeating and crowds out a desire to eat often.

Garlic — The oil of garlic contains many things — sulfides and disulfides which combat virus organisms. Garlic therapy should be started at the first hint of a sore throat or cough, which will abate the oncoming symptoms of a cold and even influenza.

Instead of submitting to the routine flu immunizing injections, why not begin each "cold season" with adding garlic capsules or perles to your diet. Or take garlic capsules or perles daily. You may find yourself not only free of colds, "flu" symptoms, sore throat, and rhinitis (clogged and running nose), but you may also discover yourself to be free of digestive problems.

Garlic perles taken with, or following, a meal equalize the acid-alkaline balance. Garlic prevents flatulence, expelling it from the stomach and intestines. The garlic oils absorbed by the mucus membranes of the stomach wall both tone and relax the stomach muscles, resulting in a natural flow of hydrochloric acid, and all the digestive fluids. The result is relief from gas pains, colic distress, belching, bloating and nausea. And, again, garlic is renowned for lowering high blood pressure.

Garlic is also renowned as a natural antibiotic. That's why it's suggested you start taking garlic oil at the first sign of flu or any virus which suggests an infection. It destroys an infection, often making it unnecessary to resort to a questionable antibiotic. It has been used as a poultice to heal skin cancer. See Chapter 11 under *Skin Cancer* for full details.

Cabbage — Cabbage is rich in calcium. Cabbage also contains a high content of phosphorus, iron, sodium and potassium. Cabbage is a sulfur food. Eat this important food once a week to avoid colon cancer. Studies show that eating cabbage not only helps prevent cancer from occurring but can even prevent the disease from spreading, if you already have it. And not just colon cancer — any cancer.

Carrots — are extremely rich in most minerals and vitamin A. One carrot a day cuts the risk of lung cancer. Carrot soup is famous in the treatment of diarrhea. The liquid content of the soup combats dehydration. It is rich in potassium, phosphorous, calcium, sulfur, magnesium and sodium, which are important to someone with diarrhea who is losing large quantities of minerals, including sodium. Carrot soup also contains pectin, so important as an antidiarrheal remedy. It coats the inflamed intestines, preventing further irritation and inflammation. Its destructive effect on undesirable intestinal bacteria prevents vomiting and, because of its effect on the peristalsis movement, it helps to eliminate toxins from the intestines.

Diluted carrot soup may be spoon-fed to infants with diarrhea or, if strained and diluted further, may be bottle fed. Carrot juice may also be bottle fed for good health in general.

An oriental method to aid digestion is to chop and dice carrots and carrot tops, place in a kettle with enough water to cover them and bring to a boil. Remove from the heat and allow to cool. Refrigerate it immediately. Strain and sip a small glass before or with each daily meal. This potion not only aids digestion but flushes the kidneys and bladder as well. And, eating plenty of carrots is also good for the complexion.

Cucumber — Sliced raw cucumbers should be added frequently to salads. It is known as a liver regenerator and an aid to digestion.

Corn — Phosphorous is abundant in corn. Corn, rich in magnesium, should be part of the diet of every cancer victim. In addition to magnesium, corn contains calcium and a rich supply of phosphoric acid. In areas where the population eats corn habitually cancer is relatively rare. Corn is rich in vitamin E. Processed cornmeal and cornstarch are degerminated foods and should be avoided. Unprocessed cornmeal may be purchased at health stores. Cornstarch should be avoided, choosing agar-agar from health stores instead.

Olive Oil and Canola Oil — All victims of hardening of the arteries should switch to the use of olive or canola oil, which are extremely rich in linoleic acid and oleic acid. Both of these natural oils help to reduce the accumulation of cholesterol in the bloodstream. When cooking with oil cannot be avoided, olive or canola oil should be selected because, due to some mysterious element, they seem not to be as affected by heat as other oils.

They are excellent sources of unsaturated fat, and people who consume them regularly seem less subject to arteriosclerosis (hardening of the arteries). These oils are preferred over other oils because of the cold processing. No chemicals are used, and no preservatives, especially olive oil from other countries.

Leeks — Leeks contain twenty-five milligrams of vitamin C in one-half cup. Leeks, like garlic, contain a substance which makes them strongly antibiotic.

Potatoes — Potatoes are rich in iron, vitamins C and B, and potassium. A medium size baked potato contains twenty milligrams of vitamin C. A medium size sweet potato contains twenty-five milligrams. Potatoes leave an alkaline ash in the stomach, reducing stomach acidity. In this sense they are much to be desired over milk, in healing ulcers for instance. There are eleven milligrams of calcium per serving.

Avoid instant mashed potatoes as the product bears little resemblance to its original name. They are loaded with preservatives, including sodium nitrate. And avoid restaurant fried potatoes, especially French fries. They have been kept in preservatives long before time for cooking and serving. To prevent the potatoes from turning black they are stored in containers filled with a solution of benzoate of soda, which is a preservative chemical you really don't need in your stomach.

If you order potato salad in a restaurant and it has a strange metallic taste do not eat it. It means it was prepared earlier in the day and stored in an aluminum container. The acidic action of the vinegar used in seasoning the salad reacts on the aluminum, absorbing much of its poison into the potatoes.

Better Butter — For those of us who love butter it's hard to resist adding it to our potatoes and vegetables. However, if you prefer the totally natural approach, fill a plastic bottle with a spout, with cold-pressed oil — such as sesame, safflower, olive, canola or almond — and drip it over your hot veggies or potatoes. Over our popcorn Robert drips olive oil. I prefer canola. Thus we avoid too much butter.

The New Pasta — White pasta, made with white flour, is usually avoided by the healthian, or held to a minimum. Available in health stores is green pasta made with spinach. Now appearing are a variety of other choices: red pasta made with flour from beets; also pink, orange, even black, all products of vegetable flours. Try them with stir-fry vegetables or baked in casseroles. Of course they contain no fat and very few calories.

Fish Warning — Just when millions were turning from beef to fish now comes a warning about a new peril — a toxic poison found in fish that feed off reefs, like red snapper, amberjack, grouper or surgeonfish. Better concentrate on deep sea fish.

Fats and Flaxseed Oil — We have already said much about flaxseed but there is more to share. We are constantly being warned to avoid fats as a part of our diet. Now we are told that there are good fats that destroy bad fats — fats that are healthy. The major good fat seems to be flaxseed oil. It seems that flaxseed oil taken daily (about 2 tablespoons) fights off the destructive effects of other oils and fats which lead to health problems such as heart disease, arteriosclerosis and degenerative conditions.

There are two essential fatty acids which the body does not manufacture within itself. They must be obtained from foods as part of the diet. They are absolutely necessary for health and even for life itself. These two fats — unsaturated linoleic and linolenic acid — are found in flaxseed oil. When shopping for flaxseed oil be sure it is cold pressed and contains a good supply of these two fatty acids. Flaxseed oil is much to be desired over fish oil in Omega-3. *Spectrum Naturals* from your health store is a good choice. It may be added to your breakfast orange juice. I also take a heaping teaspoon of flaxseed swallowed down with water twice a day. Helps me stay thin and aids in cleansing the colon.

Neutralizing Harmful Negative Energy Fields From Foods — Use Shaklee's Basic H, Amway's LOC solution, or apple cider vinegar for soaking all food. Or try *F-V Wash*. It is a product that removes up to 97% of the surface pesticides, chemicals and waxes on fruit and vegetables. It can be obtained by writing to Consumer Health Research, Inc. (Address elsewhere.) Or use Wysong's Frugie Spray from Swanson's. Follow instructions given on any of these products.

The Preparation of Foods: Avoid cooking in aluminum, even that which is coated. Avoid foods that are wrapped, canned, or packaged in aluminum foil or cans. Read labels. Avoid alum or any salt-of-aluminum fillers, puddings, pies, baked goods, pickles, most cheeses and ice cream (buy honey ice cream). Baking powder contains aluminum unless it is Rumfords. Buy fresh foods in season. Avoid canned and prepared foods. Avoid drinks in aluminum cans. Aluminum is now recognized as a causative in Alzheimer's disease.

Avoid saccharin or sucaryl. They are chemical. Do not salt your food for cooking, add it after cooking. Use Real Salt or any good mineral salt from the health store, or order mineral salt from the Dews Company. Use date sugar, raw natural honey, or pure maple sugar or syrup instead of white sugar. If date sugar is unavailable order it from Shields Date Gardens. Or order Sweet Charge from the Dews Company as a substitute for white sugar. It contains no sugar, no saccharin, no sodium and all ingredients are used by the body as food since they are all found in fresh, uncooked foods. It looks like white sugar. (All addresses in last chapter.)

Do not mix fruits with sugars or starches. Never mix meat and dairy products at the same meal. Do not eat two proteins at the same meal. Do not mix proteins with sugars and starches. Never mix acid and alkaline foods.

Those familiar with the use of a bar magnet should use the north pole of the magnet to energize food or water.

Cold processed coffee made in a Toddy coffee maker contains less caffeine and less toxic oils. Soak the filter in Clorox.

Bless your food before eating. Ask that all radiations and harmful energies be rendered harmless. To stay in good health seek out those you have hurt or wronged and ask their forgiveness.

Why I Am a Vegetarian

Most people think that the harder one labors the more meat one needs. The direct opposite is true. Meat is aging. It's toxic. And it's loaded with uric acid. Meat contains waste products that the animal would have eliminated. The flesh of the human body absorbs the waste of the meat. When these animal wastes reach the body cells they cause aging and fatigue. Principal among body waste products are urea and uric acid. Beefsteak contains about fourteen grains of uric acid per pound. When beef is boiled waste appears as a soluble extract in the form of beef broth. When analyzed it closely corresponds with urine.

Uric acid is the leading cause of arthritis. Could arthritics be victims of a carnivorous diet? Could the wastes in meat, saturating human cells, cause cancer? Or multiple sclerosis? Or Parkinson's? Or Alzheimer's? Or any of the other numerous diseases? Just a thought.

To me, meat breeds more disease in the human body

than any other food. It's well known that diseased animals are quickly sold to slaughter houses before they can die a natural death. The late Dr. John Harvey Kellogg once said when he sat down to a vegetarian dinner, "It's nice to eat a meal and not have to worry about what your food may have died from."

Meat inspectors know better than anyone about diseased meat sold for food. A story in a recent vegetarian magazine describes an actual happening. A lady attending a banquet asked if she might please have a vegetarian plate. So did the gentleman sitting next to her. "So you're a vegetarian?" he asked. "Yes," she replied, "Are you?" "No," he answered, "I'm a meat inspector." Animal diseases must surely be communicated to the persons who eat them.

You think you do better by eating fish or chicken? A scientist studying cancer in chickens wrote this in the magazine, *Poultry Science*: "The conclusions drawn must consider the possibility that many chickens show the basic microscopic lesions of lymphomatosis." That's cancer. And sad to say, most fish have worms, called anisakiasis. It's not *my* opinion. Go fishing, select a fish, split it with a sharp knife, then hold the thin section up to the light. Possibly, you'll see worms embedded in the flesh. Of course, cooking destroys the worms. But raw fish or undercooked fish can infect you with a serious illness which mimics appendicitis. You could be rushed to a hospital and booked for an unnecessary appendectomy. Avoid sushi, sashimi and all undercooked fish. Eat fish broiled, baked, poached, grilled or fried.

These are only the physical reasons I'm a vegetarian. For spiritual reasons I would be, even if the above conditions were nonexistent. To do spiritual service, such as healing, one should purify the body as much as possible. And that, above all, makes vegetarianism right and easy — and enjoyable — as a way of living. Health stores now carry excellent meat substitutes. Search for those free of monosodium glutamate and artificial flavors. Subscribe to the magazine *Vegetarian Times*, P.O. Box 446, Mount Morris, IL. 61054, for excellent sources of vegetarian food and cooking.

Chapter Eighteen

Holistic Methods to Wholeness

The principal purpose of this book is to guide the health-seeker toward alternative methods to overcome illnesses and maintain health. Therefore the writings and research would be pointless without guidelines toward such methods. That's one purpose of holistic medicine — to offer alternative choices. I hope this chapter will help you find your way through the confusion one often meets in seeking physical wholeness and well-being.

Acupinch — For sudden injury, or even for sustained pain, try pinching the upper lip between the thumb and index finger. Try it for muscle cramps. Often the pain subsides immediately.

Adrenals — Try licorice. And add vitamin C and vitamin D to your diet. Maybe there's some wisdom to the old adage "early to bed and early to rise." Certainly the early-to-bed person may never need a shot of cortisone since the body manufactures its own supply during the hours of 9:00 p.m. to 11:00 p.m. It also manufactures its own adrenaline, pepsin and insulin. The manufacturing process seems to work best if the body is bedded down and in repose. So if you go to bed early you may never have arthritis or any of the other ailments that require injections of cortisone or adrenal enforcement. Also ask your doctor or your health store concerning pantothenic acid for healing exhausted adrenals.

We hear much about the effect of stress in connection with emotional involvement, but little about its effect upon the physical body. Probably the most seriously affected are the adrenal glands. Every form of stress, whether physical or emotional, affects the adrenal glands. The raw material of the glands — which include cholesterol and ascorbic acid — are depleted and a lack of adrenal hormones result.

When the raw materials which produce the important adrenaline — hydrocortisone, pepsin and insulin — are consistently depleted, the adrenals can no longer supply the hormones necessary for well-being. The loss of adrenal hormones result in many health problems. A major function of the glands is to produce hydrocortisone. When a weakened adrenal gland fails to produce sufficient hydrocortisone the result is excessive inflammation and the appearance of arthritis, asthma and allergies of every kind.

When a doctor, after examining you, prescribes cortisone — a synthetic hormone — he is actually telling you your adrenal glands are not properly functioning. But taking injections of synthetic cortisone causes extreme side effects. It would be much wiser to reactivate your own adrenals through proper nutrition and herbs. See your therapist about a program to stimulate the adrenals or inquire concerning the *Super Adrenal Formula* by writing to BBC, address in last chapter. Or write Michael Tierra for an herbal remedy. Osteopaths often prescribe homeopathic remedies or herbs for such problems.

Practice the yogic Cobra Pose which has been described in Chapter 13 under *Sinus Congestion*.

Air Purifiers — Did you know you can purify the air in your home through certain house plants? Ivy or spider plants are good, but they must be planted in potting soil combined with activated charcoal which acts as a filter to remove or neutralize impure and polluted air.

Amino Acids — Be very sure of your daily intake of amino acids. They are excellent for pain, inflammation, and to balance the entire system. Deficiency of *threonine* causes neurologic dysfunction and pain in the joints. It also causes a deficiency in the immune system. Taking threonine stimulates the immune system which results in all manner of benefits, including balancing the thyroid gland, preventing multiple sclerosis, muscle spasms, depression, manic depression, peptic ulcer, spastic colon, and high blood pressure.

For those low in thyroid activity, iodine therapy is indicated. Kelp is an excellent source of iodine. Evening primrose oil is also indicated because it stimulates the body to produce substances similar to those of thyroid hormones.

A recent letter from one of my favorite Astarians tells me about Custer, an Indian medicine man, and what he had to say about pain and amino acids. The letter was so explicit in detail it is printed in full:

"Once a year try the following formula: mix one tablespoon of lemon juice and one of pure cold pressed virgin olive oil and take first thing in the morning — before any food is taken. Do this for twenty-one mornings. It surely cleans the liver and the gall bladder, and that seems to help everything. It will not do any good taken any other time of day.

"Now for the amino acids. I thought I had hurt my back from lifting, also thought I had arthritis in my knees, ankles and shoulders. It was very difficult to walk up steps, or to lie down and then get up. The pain was there in full force. So I went back to Custer, the Indian Medicine Man. He said I didn't hurt myself, that all I needed were amino acids, and to get them from a health food store. It worked! I am free of pain and it didn't take long.

"Also my son had a severe pain in his heart. He couldn't lie down and to use his arms was most painful. Custer also put him on amino acids. He went home and took eight amino acid caps and the next morning he felt very well. The pain had gone away! Taking eight caps of amino acids at once was unheard of, but he was desperate for relief from pain and it worked for him. The pain has not returned! It took Custer 14 years of training to become a healer and he is a great one."

Antibiotics — When a doctor prescribes antibiotics, do increase your intake of vitamin B, because antibiotics tend to create deficiencies of the B vitamins. Choose sublingual tincture. Also increase the intake of vitamin C, silica, magnesium and zinc. Also immediately begin taking acidophilus, either in pill form or through yogurt, because antibiotics also destroy friendly intestinal bacteria. With the loss of such friendly bacteria in the intestines, one could easily fall victim to candidiasis (fungus infection) either in the intestines or in the genital area.

Appendicitis — If an abdominal pain causes a suspicion of appendicitis, yet you are uncertain, here is a simple test. Standing with your knees straight, rise on your toes for a few seconds, then come down hard with your full weight on your heels. If you feel a sharp pain in the abdomen, the likelihood of appendicitis exists. If no sudden sharp pain, probably not. The jarring heel-drop test results in pain which is indicative of appendicitis. The test is quick and costs nothing to perform. But for certain diagnosis see your doctor.

Asthma — is often caused by food allergies. Try adding boiled carrots to the diet to eliminate allergy-related substances from the body. Also drop five drops of cold pressed castor oil under the tongue daily.

Aerobic exercises can prevent asthma attacks. They increase the lungs' ability to use oxygen. Be sure to perform warm-up exercises a few moments before beginning aerobics. Start slowly and work up to more vigorous routines. End with more simple exercises. Be sure to have a bronchodilator handy in case it's needed.

Many asthma and emphysema sufferers claim they receive relief by sniffing Chihuahuas. Though experts cannot explain it, most asthma and emphysema patients who have tried it insist they feel much better after a good whiff of the coats of the little Mexican pups.

Bar Magnets — can be used to destroy infections, reduce inflammation, reduce pain and stimulate the thyroid. Do study literature concerning the north and south poles of the magnets, and hold them over the problem areas. See Chapter 9 for more information or write to Bio Health Enterprises, Inc. See the last chapter for address.

The Health Bath

Many have written offering suggestions about bath soaks that cleanse the body of toxins, beautify the skin, and remove aches and pains — and radiation from x-rays, as well. All of these are 20-minute soaks. Water should be only slightly warmer than tepid. Bath water too hot draws energy from the body and is not wise. Herbal oils or powders should be added to replenish the natural skin oils, or applied to the body after the bath. A plain tub bath dries the skin.* After each soak be sure to rinse your body by showering to remove toxins which have surfaced during the soak. Either bath or shower should include a friction rub. A mitt glove containing wet bristles is excellent. The friction brushes away many dead cells and increases circulation on the surface of the skin. Occasionally when showering sponge your body with Epsom salts water — one teaspoon of Epsom salts in two cups of warm water. Dip the sponge mitt in this solution to sponge off dead cells and toxins.

The Clorox Bath — Add seven ounces of liquid regular unscented Clorox to a tub of water. Rub the skin thoroughly with a rough washcloth or loofah brush during the soak. After the soak shower thoroughly to destroy an odor of Clorox. Some suggest drinking a glass of water with five drops of Clorox while soaking. Many people while traveling in foreign countries take Clorox along and add some to their drinking water to remove substances which could cause tummy upsets.

Epsom Salts/Peroxide Bath — Add one pint of 3% hydrogen peroxide, available at the drug store, and two cups of Epsom salts to a full tub of water. A 20-minute soak will ease aches and pains and leave the skin in good tone.

Mineral Tub Soak — There's nothing like having a mineral bath in your own tub. Add Earth Force Minerals to your 20-minute soak. Some people claim cures for arthritis and all manner of other problems. For information

*See *Forever Young.*

about this amazing product write B&K Products. (See last chapter for address.)

Skin Cleanser — Many toxins are eliminated through the pores. To remove any contamination and bacteria or simply to cleanse the skin, mix five pints of 3% hydrogen peroxide to two pints of Aloe Vera juice with one pint of glycerin. Add a cup of this formula to your bath soak, or sponge off the body using this solution.

Oak Bark Skin Cleanser — To a full tub add a squirt of Fanie's Oak Bark Skin Cleanser or Sweet Birch Bath Cleanser.

The Tea Tree Bath — For muscle aches rub pure Tea Tree Oil directly into the muscles. And add ten drops to a hot tub and soak.

The White Vinegar Bath — Add a cup or two of white vinegar to a tub of water for muscle and heel pains. Never use apple cider vinegar in a tub soak. Never allow apple cider vinegar to enter the vagina. It could trigger yeast infection. Use only white vinegar in a douche. One teaspoon to a quart.

Baths to Counteract X-Ray and Radiation — Vitamin B6, taken daily, will help your body expel the effects of radiation and x-ray. Also vitamin C. Many holistic doctors suggest soaking in a warm tub bath with two cups of Epsom salts and two cups of baking soda added to counteract the radiation. Repeat twice a week for a month. Drink a cup of chamomile tea while soaking. The tea opens the pores to release toxins stored in tissues and muscles so shower afterward.

Bed Sores — For a patient enduring a long stay in bed add sublingual vitamin B to the diet to avoid the development of bed sores. A body rub with castor oil is most healing. Also Tea Tree Oil.

Biomagnetic Bracelets — Biomagnetic bracelets have become extremely popular in Europe. The bracelet is copper dipped in gold. It is embedded with magnets. They are said to alter the regulation of biomagnetic energies to discharge static electricity and void an overcharge of positive ions. Eventually they improve the circulation and balance the nervous system. The late Dr. Ralph Sierra, a world pioneer in the study of magnetic healing, is credited with saving the health of many sportsmen, actors, actresses and others seeking muscle and bone healing through applied magnets.

Biorhythms — Most of us have long suspected that our lives are influenced by certain cycles. But until biorhythms came on the scene the cycles were not clearly marked out for us in a practical manner — that is, via a chart that might be studied and made applicable in daily use. Biorhythm research has produced the theory that, beginning at the moment of birth, all human lives move in three predictable cycles: a physical cycle of 23 days, an emotional cycle of 28 days and an intellectual cycle of 33 days. In each cycle, half the days are plus and half are minus.

In the 23 day *physical cycle*, the 11 1/2 plus days are a good time for any activity requiring physical stamina. During the 11 1/2 minus days, one should be aware that he/she is in a low cycle of reduced vitality and endurance. Illness is not indicated by any means, simply that you are not at your physical best and may tire more easily.

The 28 day cycle, the *emotional cycle*, corresponds approximately to the lunar month which involves a woman's menstrual cycle. But men are also involved. During the 14 plus days, both men and women experience a sense of well-being, happiness, and a positive attitude toward life. For both, the 14 minus days are prone to negativism, depression, low moods.

During the 16 1/2 plus days of the *intellectual cycle* the creative forces are flowing. The mind is alert and receptive to an inflow of ideas. The writer is more creative, the student is more alert, the housewife is in full control of planning, the secretary is more efficient, the executive is extremely productive. In every avenue the mind is open to learn more and retain more. In the 16 1/2 minus days one should not push toward one's best creative efforts. This is the time to mentally coast, putting into practice that which was learned during the plus cycle or reviewing creative endeavors.

The day the cycle changes from plus to minus or from minus to plus is recognized as a critical day. This is true of all three cycles. This switch-over day is called a zero day. You are in a state of limbo, your worst possible time. You are neither up nor down. You aren't in full control. You should be aware you are neither plus nor minus.

In the *physical cycle* the critical day is when people are accident prone. On the critical day of the *emotional cycle* one is subject to possible emotional outbursts. In the *intellectual cycle* the critical day is not so obvious unless it happens to coincide with a critical day of another cycle. The day or days when all three cycles are simultaneously critical, it would be far wiser simply to "stay in bed" — at least it is wise to be totally aware that you are in a cycle of nonproductiveness, that you are accident prone and you are subject to simultaneous emotional outbursts. You are not in full control.

Research clearly shows that accident case histories reported by insurance companies are definitely related to zero points on a biorhythm chart. Physical or emotional zero days occur on an average of one day out of six and double zero days about six times a year. Triple zero days — when your physical, emotional and intellectual cycles are combined in their switch-over point — occur only about once a year.

There is also reason for caution when you are at the peak of a physical cycle while experiencing zero in your emotional and intellectual days. This would indicate your sense of physical well-being might cause you to overlook obvious dangers and become ripe for an accident.

Although the biorhythm theory has not been scientifically proven, the 28 day menstrual cycle for the female is closely tied in with the biorhythm 28 day emotional cycle, and although men experience no menstrual cycle they obviously respond to a fluctuating emotional cycle.

Industry is now slowly becoming aware of the possibilities of these three biorhythmic theories. Air industries are beginning to chart their pilots. Bus companies are charting the work days of their drivers. In Switzerland doctors are beginning to use the theory to discover the best day for surgical operations. As usual the United States lags far behind in applying the theory to industry or medicine. As in astrology, one need not base one's entire life and decisions on one's biorhythm charts. It is only meant that one should be aware of the possibilities involved.

Bleeding — For excessive bleeding dip sterile cotton into hot water and press it on the wound until the bleeding stops.

Breath Healing — Yogic breathing exercises aid complete elimination of poisons through the lungs, the breath and the complete respiratory tract.* Next time you visit

*See *The Book of Beginning Again*.

your doctor for your annual checkup ask him to add the *spirometer test* to his routine. It's as important as a blood pressure test but is usually neglected. All you have to do is inhale and exhale into a tube to check your lung capacity. Simple as it is, it reveals any impaired lung function which could warn whether or not you're a candidate for a stroke or heart attack.

If you have a lung problem — asthma, emphysema, chronic bronchitis, tuberculosis, cancer, or any other breathing difficulty — do be aware of a new hot line created just to give you further information and guidelines. It's located in Denver, Colorado. See last chapter for the telephone number.

Burns — For minor burns and sunburn flush first with cold water/ice pack immediately. Then apply Tea Tree Oil directly to the burn. See section on Tea Tree Oil later on in this chapter for further information regarding this miraculous natural remedy.

Testing Your Calcium Tablet — Many take wrong calcium tablets, unaware that the body is not being properly supplemented. To test your calcium tablet drop one in a glass of white or apple cider vinegar. It should dissolve into fine particles within thirty minutes. If it does not switch to another brand of calcium supplements. Researchers are now beginning to believe the very best source of calcium is through silica — silica and magnesium. "They" say that taking calcium tablets often causes arthritis, inflammation and calcified deposits throughout the body. Since reading these reports, I've given up calcium for silica and magnesium. Already my nails and hair are responding.

Chamomile Herbal Products to the Rescue — When Dr. Som lived one of his principal cures for almost everything was chamomile herbal products. Today it seems to be enjoying recognition throughout the health field. It's now being used as a mouth and throat spray, as a hair rinse to highlight the hair, as a pain relieving cream to bring relief of minor pain in muscles and joints, arthritis pains, backaches, and bruises. It's also used for skin irritation and as a substitute for any problems requiring corticosteroids. Chamomile Cream and chamomile capsules are available at your health store.

Castor Oil — Rub on soles of feet. For hyperactive children: five drops a day in juice or honey, or dropped directly under the tongue to heal allergies and other problems. For arthritis: garlic, turmeric, red pepper cooked in castor oil, strained and rubbed on joints. Rub castor oil on back of neck to restore gray hair; soaked tampon in rectum or vagina for any genital problem; rubbed on Herpes Zoster; oil mixed with Aloe Vera for ulcers. Rub on itching skin; rub on lower abdomen each night to help correct constipation, to heal adhesions, to correct other "inner" problems. Use only cold pressed oil, available from Cayce Corner. (Address elsewhere.) For eyes apply a poultice of cotton pats dipped in chamomile tea with drops of cold pressed castor oil and raw honey added.

Castor Oil Packs — acclaimed by the A.R.E. folks (Edgar Cayce), have constantly proven to be highly effective in stimulating the immune system. The castor oil pack is nothing more than a cotton flannel cloth drenched in cold pressed castor oil and placed upon the lower abdomen preferably at bedtime. The oil should also be massaged into the abdomen. If the pack proves too troublesome just apply castor oil directly on the abdomen. Such a simple treatment as a castor oil pack is effective for many purposes — constipation, tennis elbow, inflamed knee joints, aching backs. The benefits are endless. Again, order cold pressed oil from Cayce Corner. (Address elsewhere.)

Chelation Therapy — Chelation therapy is an alternate approach to cleaning debris from your arteries to avoid a heart attack, or to maintain clean arteries after an attack. An artificial amino acid called EDTA (ethylene-diamine-tetra-acetate acidic acid) is fed intravenously into the bloodstream, along with vitamin-mineral supplements, for the purpose of breaking up calcified deposits along the walls of the arteries. This EDTA "captures" these plaque fragments, together with metal found floating in the blood, and carries them out of the body via the systems of elimination.

Although this modality is often decried by the conventional medic, its success is widely noted. The usual medical approach offers little to help except drastic surgery, and still heart disease ranks as our number one killer. Chelation offers a "natural" approach, considerably cheaper and with little risk. One *can* obtain oral chelation through herbal methods, but it's a slower process, requiring approximately a year and a half for effective results. Hanna Kroeger's *Circu-Flow* is excellent. And Michael Tierra offers an excellent herbal chelation. Contact him for information.

The benefits of EDTA chelation therapy can no longer be denied. Too many patients have made spectacular improvements. The only group vociferously opposed seems to be the medical practitioners who have no personal experience with the therapy and who refuse to consider the records established by those who have. Intravenous EDTA, as stated, removes metals from the bloodstream which in itself is enough to applaud the therapy, because it thus eliminates a biochemical cause of aging and prevents damage to cells and enzymes. Of course it must be given according to established guidelines, nor does anyone claim it to be an all inclusive treatment in the prevention of heart problems. Diet, as is obvious, is extremely important in any disease, but especially that of the heart. But anyone experiencing heart problems should most certainly consider chelation therapy, which requires a change in diet.

Choking — Should you begin choking on food when you are alone do get your feet higher than your head. Lie on a bed with your head on the floor face down, or across a chair. Or lie face down on stairs with your head downward. Gravity has been known to release stuck food.

Colostrum Cream or Tablets — Colostrum is the substance obtained during the first few days after parturition. It's source is mother's milk. This special fluid — the first milk secreted by the mammary glands immediately after childbirth — is very rich in immune factors. The presence of colostrum the first few days after birth is the major reason doctors prefer mothers to breast feed their babies. Colostrum contains every known factor for providing the newborn with every possible protection against diseases or infections. It contains 55% immunoglobulins, antibody stimulating factors, hormones, vitamins, nucleotides, enzymes and various nonimmunal globulin components that destroy microcosms which could cause disease.

The benefits of colostrum in cream form and taken in capsules reads like a miracle report. The cream not only removes wrinkles and restores youth to the face, but it also heals all manner of skin problems, including serious burns. Taken in capsule form it is a direct immunal stimulant which aids the body in restoring itself to total and complete health.

Colostrum has been shown to be of supreme benefit to

people experiencing stiff, swollen joints, which could be the result of infection in other areas of the body, or a reaction to an allergy. Do consider colostrum if you are in any way immobilized with painful joints. Both the cream and the tablets may be ordered from Dr. Charles W. Bunner (address elsewhere). Dr. Bunner declares that he has seen it perform miracles, not only with sore and painful arthritic joints but in abscesses, severe headaches, tumors, toothaches and deafness.

Corns — Try a slice of lemon fastened on the corn overnight, or soak your feet in warm water and baking soda for 30 minutes. The soda dissolves the hard corn.

Diabetes — Dr. P. Ebeling of The National Public Health Institute in Finland, reports that a long-term, moderate supplementation of *guar gum* improves the meal tolerance and glycemic control of diabetics. Research at Helsinki University showed that after one month of taking 5g. guar gum four times a day before meals, Type I diabetics had considerable lower blood glucose levels, their serum total cholesterol dropped 21%, and they needed 5% less insulin. Guar gum tablets are available at your health store. Or order from Swanson.

Olive oil in the diet also helps lower the blood sugar levels of most adult-onset diabetes and reduces the daily insulin needs. It also reduces blood levels of triglycerides. The combination of these benefits could help prevent some of the more serious complications of diabetes. And if you don't like olive oil you could substitute another oil high in monounsaturated fats such as peanut oil or canola oil.

Dieting — If you are trying to lose weight here's a happy, helpful hint. Try painting your dining area light blue or light green. Or simply add splashes of these colors to your surroundings. Studies have shown that light blue and green can help suppress your appetite. Stay away from orange, red or yellow. These colors stimulate the appetite.

Diverticulitis — Try the homeopathic remedy called *Mag Phos*.

DMSO — Americans are sometimes told that DMSO is not only noneffective but inadvisable. However, in 1808 Russian lumberjacks, working in below freezing weather, discovered that if they rubbed DMSO (a product of natural tree bark) on their aching joints, the pain would quickly depart — and so would swollen arthritis joints. More recently its entire history is beneficial. If not, I wonder why horse breeders use it persistently on their lame and crippled horses?

Drug Addiction — Drug addicts would do well to add silica to the diet. There is a toll-free hot line number in the last chapter for help with drug problems.

Ears

Earache — After each haircut, be sure loose hair is washed from the ears with the next shampoo. If left in the ear a blow dryer could blow the hair deep inside the ear causing severe pain.

When we were young Mama used to put sweet oil in our aching ears. Sweet oil is a refined olive oil from drug stores. If the child still pulls or rubs the ear see a doctor immediately. An untreated ear infection can lead to serious complications. The infection can spread to other head centers causing loss of hearing and impaired speech development. Now the usual treatment is penicillin, but many react to penicillin. If you cannot take penicillin because of allergic reaction try the homeopathic remedy called *Ferrum Phosphoricum*.

To help prevent earache keep the ears warm in cold weather, even with earmuffs. Keep water out of the ears. Wear molded earplugs when swimming or showering. Bottle feed babies in an upright position, never while lying flat. If there is pain apply heat. Never dig into the ear with a toothpick, hairpin, cotton swab, or anything else attempting to remove wax. See a doctor. Inquire from Michael Tierra or Hanna Kroeger concerning the best herbal approach. Hanna's product *Tune In* to improve memory also improves hearing.

Ringing in Ears — avoid loud noises; avoid caffeine and other stimulants. Exercise; get plenty of rest; meditate to reduce stress. Toss away your refined white table salt, which impairs circulation, and buy mineral salt from your health store, or order mineralized salt from the Dews Co. Consider removing the silver fillings in your teeth. Their removal has been known to terminate this problem. There is a new product that is getting rave reviews from its users. Its name is *Tinnitus Relief* and its ingredients are all natural. It's worth a try. From your health store or call 1-800-221-1152.

Epileptic Seizures — The usual medical procedure is to give Phenobarbital and Dilantin and dismiss the patient to his own fate. The only hope is to try a cleansing diet of raw food — fruits, vegetables, herb teas and massive doses of vitamin C. Add vitamin B6 to the diet. Also watermelon. Make sure the bowels are open even if enemas are temporarily required. Avoid homogenized cow's milk. Try raw whole milk, or raw goat's milk. You may wish to have your silver dental fillings removed. See Chapter 15. Write Hanna Kroeger or Michael Tierra for herbal help.

The Importance of Exercise — To maintain good well-being and an active immune system exercise is mandatory.

Women who do not exercise run twice the risk of developing cancer in the reproductive system and breasts. Also, exercise seems to prevent cancer of the colon. Exercise also builds the immune system to fight off colds, flu and other infections. It overcomes insomnia, relieves depression and even helps to keep the body youthful. Try walking. Try riding a stationary bicycle. Try the isometric exercises given in *The Book of Beginning Again*. Try the yogic technique of Salutation to the Sun.

Eyes

Bloodshot Eyes — For bloodshot eyes try putting a drop of raw castor oil into the eye.

Contact Lenses — There are now disposable contact lenses designed to be worn continuously for about a week and then discarded. They are called *Acuvue*. These disposable lenses reduce the possibility of infection, which can occur with the extended wearing of soft contact lenses.

Electroretinogram — is a device that measures the eye's response to visual stimuli. It may also be used to detect the approach of Alzheimer's, glaucoma and diabetic retinopathy long before they are diagnosed. It's known as *pr-ERG*.

Eye Drops — A health letter released by the Mayo Clinic states that prescription eye drops can cause changes in emotions and behavior and affect organs far away from the eyes. The drops are those that are prescribed to widen or narrow the pupil, change lens curvature or reduce fluid pressure. But they also affect the autonomic nervous system which controls heart rate, blood pressure and vital functions of the lungs, bladder, stomach and intestinal tract. The drops may also alter brain chemicals, affecting thought processes. Check with your doctor.

Eyes and Diet — Glutathione, a protein found in green leafy vegetables, is proving beneficial in protecting the retina against the damaging effect of ultraviolet rays. Also vitamin E. Those with glaucoma should never drink over 2 cups of coffee a day. Caffeine increases the pressure in the eye.

Dangers of Fluorescent Lighting — It is well known that fluorescent lighting damages the eyesight. Those who are concerned should know about Kiva-Light, a full spectrum light, whose bulbs and tubes fit normal lighting fixtures and provide light similar to that of the sun. Or the full spectrum light tubes sold by John Ott. It is important, not only for our eyesight, but for our general health, always to use full spectrum light. Kiva-Light and John Ott offer the only full spectrum lighting tubes of which I am aware. Do substitute your fluorescent tubes for either of these. Order from L.O. Anderson Research Laboratory or directly from Ott Light Systems, Inc. (See last chapter for addresses).

Massage Technique for Improved Eyesight — Vision Improvement Centers Inc. of Calgary, Alberta, Canada, is the first research center in North America to begin using a Japanese computer-controlled massage technique to improve eyesight. The technique employs a shiatsu therapeutic massage using a computer rather than human hands to stimulate centers which correct vision impairment. The Japanese hope the technique will soon be available in our U.S.

Miracle Specs — are sometimes called stress specs. They look like regular sun glasses except that they have liquid crystals attached to the inside of each lens. The glasses are worn whenever pain is present. They are effective in releasing tension which causes tension headaches, lowering high blood pressure and relieving insomnia. Ask your doctor for information concerning these stress specs if you suffer from any of the above problems.

Removing an Object From the Eye — First wash your hands. Don't rub. Blink repeatedly to produce tears. Use an eyedropper containing contact lens solution, eye-wash, or even water to flush out object. Pull down lower lid and with a clean tissue gently try to flick out object. If it's under the upper lid gently grasp the upper lashes between thumb and forefinger and lift the lid out and down over lower lid. The speck usually will stick to the lower lid where it can be brushed away. If all fails see an eye doctor immediately.

Fever — is the sign that nature is producing a cure and, if left alone, will do its part in curing, after which it subsides. Any measure, any medicine, that kills nature's power to produce a fever could very possibly kill the sick person. Even Hippocrates said, "Give me fever and I can cure any disease." It is usually a mistake to take a drug to bring down a fever, since fever is nature's way of burning out impurities in the body.

When a fever develops it indicates that all other avenues of elimination are clogged, and the impurities cannot escape any other way except to burn their way to the surface of the skin in the form of a fever. So the first thing to do is help nature eliminate poison through natural channels by taking an enema twice daily. Often the fever will immediately break.

Make sure the bowels stay open. Drink watermelon seed tea or blessed thistle tea to stimulate the kidneys. Begin taking vitamin C tablets in massive doses to help fight the infection somewhere in the body (1000 mg. per hour). Since vitamin C causes the heart to beat faster during a disease crisis, keep the heart under control by taking cayenne herbal capsules, which are also excellent for burning out the infection. But take the cayenne only with food. Sensitive empty stomachs sometimes react. Or take goldenseal herbal capsules.

Take garlic perles, which are also antibiotic and help to kill germs, bacteria and virus infection. Sponge the body with cool water. Stop all foods except fruit and vegetable juices, except a small amount taken with the cayenne capsules.

Fingernail Infections — For infections in the fingernail or toenails soak nail in pure Tea Tree Oil for five minutes and massage in twice daily until the infection is gone. A word of warning to women who wear acrylic nails: they can destroy your real nails. Your nails can become disfigured, develop infections, or even fall out. If you *must* occasionally wear false nails wear the press-on kind.

Hiccups — Try crushed pineapple; or a teaspoon of peanut butter; or a small dish of ice cream; or a tablespoon of granulated sugar, chewed slowly and allowed to gradually mix with saliva. None of these should be taken with liquids. Rub the earlobes with your thumb and forefinger for several minutes. Or rub the roof of your mouth gently. Try angostura bitters on a wedge of lime. Pour a few drops of bitters on the lime wedge. Bite the lime wedge making sure the bitters and pulp of the lime are consumed.

Hyperbaric Oxygen Therapy — Hyperbaric oxygen therapy or HBO, as it is called, is one of the most wonderful new age modalities to happen for those truly searching for a holistic approach to health. It's a chamber eight feet long and three feet in diameter. You, as a patient, enter the chamber, lie down full length for a couple of hours, and emerge from the glass covered "cocoon" energized. It's wired for sound and you can communicate with a nearby technician.

The treatment consists of intermittent exposure of the entire body to 100% oxygen at above normal atmospheric pressures. It floods the body tissues with oxygen. It is excellent for treating circulation problems, healing radiation damage from cancer treatment, and healing ulcers or wounds that otherwise stubbornly will not heal.

Everyone knows the necessity of oxygen but few realize how starved the cells get as one ages. This "chamber" therapy stimulates white blood cell activity, thus preventing infections. It increases circulation by enhancing new blood vessel growth. It expands arteries, relieving blockages. It increases oxygen flow to muscles. No needles, no pills, no x-rays, no radiation, nothing but just good oxygen, hopefully the way God made it. You just lie there and breathe. Michael Jackson, the famous pop star, has made the chamber equally famous. He owns one and sleeps in it. Don't think it's bizarre. It's one of the greatest healing devices ever made. If I had a spare $90,000, I'd certainly buy one — and sleep in it!

Immunity Boosters — Gerovital (GH3) has been mentioned as a great immunity booster. Also Q10. (See *Forever Young*) Now comes word that vitamin E has proven effective in helping the elderly fight off diseases. It, too, stimulates the response of white blood cells to fight invading substances.

And aspirin! I must reluctantly report it, too, has been found extremely effective. It helps prevent heart attacks, shields against a second attack, aids pregnant mothers to bear healthier babies, increases two of the body's own infection-fighting biochemicals — interferon and interleukin-2 — and helps women undergoing radiation therapy for breast cancer return to immune status sooner than those who didn't take aspirin.

It boosts the immune system to ward off colds. People taking daily aspirin seldom get colds, say the researchers at George Washington University. Taken with DLPA (an amino acid available from health stores) for seven days straight, it's supposed to build up a tremendous immunity against pain. Where once, with me, this little white pill couldn't get any respect, it's about to take a place of honor on my "pill shelf." Increase your vitamin C intake when and if you take aspirin daily. It leaches vitamin C from the system.

Inflammation — Take massive doses of vitamin C, up to 1,000 milligrams per hour. Decrease dosage after three days.

Kelp — Those who must avoid a "pure" form of table salt may find kelp powder a welcome addition to their diet. Use it to replace salt. Kelp tablets help prevent iodine deficiencies and may aid in reducing menopausal symptoms, such as hot flashes. And of course you have already read in Chapter 9 how effective it is in treating thyroid imbalances. Kelp has also been found to prevent the absorption of metals, such as lead, in your system. Sounds like a good source of natural chelation therapy, doesn't it? Sprinkle it on foods in the place of salt and certainly over your soups and salads. Or take a kelp tablet daily.

Laughter & Healing — We've all read the story of how laughing can heal most any illness. We've usually attributed it to simply a change in conscious awareness and attitude but there seems to be also a physical cause. We know now that laughter stimulates the production of alertness hormones called *catecholamines*. These, in turn, release endorphins, which we know to be the brain's natural pain killers. Once these endorphins are released and the patient becomes more relaxed and free of pain, a sense of well-being and relaxation is experienced — a type of euphoria. Laughter also increases energy. It takes the mind off the disability problem, causing the immune system to be stimulated in a subconscious effort to fight off the illness.

Hospitals are now beginning to provide humor rooms for patients. These contain books of humorous nature and VCR comedy movies on television sets, which have recorded the funny episodes once seen on film in earlier days of movie making. There should be humor rooms in all hospitals, featuring old runs of Candid Camera, Laurel and Hardy, Charlie Chaplin, Harold Lloyd, the Three Stooges, the Marx Brothers, Bill Cosby, Jackie Gleason and Art Carney, Lucille Ball, Abbott and Costello, and all manner of other old comedies.

We all know the story of Norman Cousins, who was stricken with a progressive crippling spinal disease called ankylosis spondylitis. For lack of something better to do, he found himself tuning in to funny programs on the television and reading funny literature. He literally laughed himself well. His recovery, he declares, was aided by the self-prescribed daily doses of humor. Proverbs 17:22 — "a merry heart doeth good like a medicine." It is well to consider how effective the biblical proverb can be.

Cousins reported in his best selling book, *Anatomy of an Illness*, that just twenty minutes of hearty laughing brought him two hours of painless sleep, and medical tests revealed that after each laugh session his crippling inflammation subsided a little more — until his disease simply vanished. It might be well to combine the usual coffee break with humor. Perhaps a wise employer should provide the coffee lounge with joke books, funny tapes and old-time movies.

At Oregon Health Sciences University, members of a local group known as *Nurses For Laughter* wear buttons that read: "Warning: Humor may be hazardous to your illness." In some hospitals cancer patients are participating in laughter therapy groups that ease the anxiety of the disease and hopefully foster recovery. Since attitude is extremely important everything should be done to create humorous situations.

We've all begun to realize cut flowers can be a detriment to healing. If a loved one enters the hospital why not send a funny book of some kind or a funny novel rather than flowers? A book of jokes would be a splendid gift. Who needs chocolate candy at a time like that? (Or any other time for that matter!)

Leg Cramps — Silica and magnesium capsules are helpful. Also vitamin B6. Potassium is often needed. Eat a lot of apples or take the vinegar-honey cocktail described elsewhere in this chapter. You may also need extra vitamin E. Try the homeopathic remedy called *Mag Phos*. Try Acupinch — pinching the upper lip between the thumb and index finger.

LSD — If you have taken LSD and are still experiencing frequent or infrequent cycles of depression and mental problems, try drinking chaparral tea. Chaparral may be taken as a tea or herb capsules, obtainable from your health store.

Lupus — is a strange malady. It's an inflammation of the skin, kidneys and heart, brought on by the body's own immune system attacking its own cells. The attack also produces arthritis, anemia and pleurisy. A "butterfly rash" across the nose signals the approach of the disease. It often goes into remission for long periods. Medications such as *Prednisone* are effective but have dreadful side effects. Could this mysterious illness be triggered by mercury leaking from silver dental fillings? Just a thought. Wouldn't hurt to have the fillings removed and see what happens. For proper removal see Chapter 15.

Measles — is a contagious disease, which means the germs are in the atmosphere. But they need not get a foothold in your body unless you provide the proper toxic environment for them. Use the same healing methods as in a common cold. Once measles are indicated you should do all possible to help break out the skin so that the toxins can more quickly escape. Saffron tea taken warm (never boil) will help the measles fully to break out. Enemas should be taken to keep the fever down and to wash poisons and toxins from the body. Coffee enemas are preferable. Three cups of lukewarm strong black coffee in an enema bag. It's advisable to lie on your right side and try to retain it for fifteen minutes before expelling.

Boil a grapefruit with its rind, strain it and drink it with a bit of honey added. Also drink alfalfa mint tea. Soak in a warm tub bath with two cups of soda added to help alkalize the skin. Take vitamin C, garlic capsules, and Propolis capsules. Eat very little food and drink a lot of liquids.

Medications by Oral Absorption — We've all experienced immediate absorption into the body through injection which distributes medication directly into the bloodstream. But we are now beginning to be offered rapid introduction by oral absorption: which means a quick spray, or dropping a few drops of a tincture under the tongue. All of us are familiar with the distribution of nitroglycerin directly under the tongue of a heart patient because, being so administered, it aids the patient immediately. The same is true of many of the health items now available in tincture form for oral absorption under the tongue. Many are available at your health store.

Lapacho Mist — is another tincture now available. It's another of those heal-all herbs from Brazilian rain forests. Sprayed under the tongue it is quickly absorbed into the bloodstream. It contains no fillers, no alcohol. It does contain the famous Taheebo (Pau D'arco) herb concentrate with vitamin C, E and selenium added. It's probably available from your health store, or contact Michael Tierra.

Memory — When the memory begins to fail add vitamin B1 to the diet. Also order an herbal product called *Tune In* from Hanna. Hanna tells me *Tune In* frequently improves the hearing as an added bonus. Or contact Michael Tierra who offers many products from rain forests all over the world. More about Hanna Kroeger and Michael Tierra in the last chapter.

Multiple Sclerosis — Dr. Som claimed he could cure multiple sclerosis through nutrition. He changed his patients immediately to a raw food diet. They ate nothing cooked. Food had to be straight from the way nature made it, including fruits, vegetables, nuts, seeds, and a few dairy products such as raw whole milk, raw unsalted butter, and natural uncooked cheese and yogurt. The only cooked foods given were grains and soy meat substitutes such as tofu, usually baked. The vitamin therapy included a vitamin-mineral supplement tablet with additional vitamin B-Complex, niacin, vitamin C, vitamin E, silica, magnesium, and folic acid.

He gave four capsules daily of an herbal parasite formula. I don't remember the name of it — but both Michael and Hanna sell excellent parasite herbal remedies. In addition, he gave six capsules daily of Jason Winter's herb formula, Zion, from any health store. Drink at least a pint of raw vegetable juice daily including carrot and celery, and a pint of fruit juices. Alternate vegetable and fruit juices. And drink an ounce of raw beet juice twice a week. Massage the body daily using sesame oil. I did not follow through on any of his patients to discover if he *did* cure the disease. I offer it only as an experiment to try. *Certainly patients with MS have recovered after having their silver dental fillings removed.* The recovery is astonishing and rapid. Do consider it.

Muscle Aches and Sprains — Soak the sprained area in warm Epsom salt water twenty minutes at a time several times a day. Rest the area. Elevate it if possible. After the soak rub pure Tea Tree Oil into sore muscle and on a sprain. Also add 10 drops to a warm bath and soak in it. See "Tea Tree Oil" in this chapter for information on how to obtain Tea Tree Oil.

Parasitic Infections — Once parasitic infections were thought to be prevalent only in underdeveloped or primitive areas. But world travel has caused exposure throughout the USA, Europe, Africa, Asia and the Orient. Some are easily recognized as tapeworms. Others are so exotic as to be unrecognizable. The parasitic infections are known as trichinosis, trichuriasis, filariasis, ascariasis, hookworm and herpes II.

Effective against such infections is garlic, now available in odorless liquid form, cayenne capsule (red pepper), wormwood, and other herbs. Write Hanna Kroeger or Michael Tierra for information concerning their parasite herbal cures. Do, too, be sure your diet includes vitamins A, B1, B2, biotin, and folic acid.

Pneumonia — is still a formidable illness because the bacteria causing it has become resistant to our present antibiotics. Air pollution is weakening our lungs. Prevention through a purified diet and exercise is still the best policy. Consider coffee enemas. Be sure to add acidophilus to your diet to offset the effect of the antibiotics. And lots of garlic. Cayce's inhalant products. Lemon water.

Poison Oak or Poison Ivy — Vitamin C is a tremendous aid. Rub with cold pressed castor oil.

Potassium Deficiency — If you are suffering from a mysterious lack of energy, or if you are being treated for high blood pressure with diuretics and you seem to be experiencing extreme weakness, have your doctor check for potassium deficiency. Diuretics remove salt and fluid from the body and, in doing so, they also remove potassium. Potassium deficiency can cause extreme tiredness, leg cramps, and heart beat irregularities — it can mimic a heart problem. Unless a doctor tests for potassium deficiency you may be taking heart medicine through a wrong diagnosis. Your doctor can prescribe potassium supplements. They are also available at your health store.

Or you may wish to begin taking apple cider vinegar-honey drinks. Two teaspoons of apple cider vinegar mixed with two teaspoons of raw honey in a cup of water can quickly raise your potassium level. This would be an ongoing treatment, of course. You should also include bananas and oranges in your diet because they are rich in potassium.

Schizophrenia — is a long-term biochemical dysfunction. Which means its deficiency lies in the body and not in the mind. Niacin (vitamin B3) has been known to produce amazing improvement. Niacin usually produces a vasodilation or flush which can often be unpleasant and could last for several hours. If such is the case switch to niacinamide, a form of vitamin B3 which does not produce vasodilation. Consider removing silver dental fillings, which certainly can cause a long-term biochemical dysfunction.

Selenium — High levels are as dangerous as low levels, each of which could cause cancer. Some, due to recent media exposure, tend to overdose which could overheat the body meridians causing a serious imbalance. Do restrict to a reasonable intake.

Shingles — A simple home remedy suggested by Dr. Robert King, professor of neurologic surgery at New York State University, says you can get up to 10 hours of relief from shingles by crushing 2 aspirin into 2 tablespoons of nail polish remover and patting the paste on the affected area with a pure cotton ball. Also try Willard Water from health stores — drink it and massage it into affected areas.

Skin Blemishes — To make your skin look great and feel great, too, make a paste of brewer's yeast and water. Apply it to your face and keep it on for one hour. Then wash it off with water.

Smog — contains ozone and nitrogen oxides, two deadly toxins. Not only is the human race affected directly but also vegetation (food crops) and our forests. The hazards of smog pollution are well known. Antioxidants are surely indicated, such as vitamin A, C and E. The amino acid L-cysteine is important. So is superoxide dismutase (SOD) and selenium.

The Clean Air Act was established in 1987 as a deadline for reducing ozone levels in our nation. A law was also passed affecting the smog produced by buses and trucks, the principal offenders. But since the law seems to have been totally ignored by these particular offenders, we have no choice but to fight, to the best of our ability, the perils that smog produces. Ask at your health store for the best antioxidants.

Soda Pop — Too much soda pop or soft drink, and in some cases, even a relatively small amount, seems to trigger behavioral problems in some children. The caffeine in soft drinks has an adverse effect on some — and combined with the sugar in it, it can cause a generally well-behaved youngster to become quite difficult to handle. The child seems to lose all self-control, is unable to sit still, and can exhibit violent behavior. So, if your youngster sometimes acts like an over-wound clock, take notice whether he or she has recently consumed a soft drink containing caffeine and/or anything with a highly concentrated amount of sugar, or a "harmless drug." It could mean a great deal to the entire family, especially to the child.

Sore Mouth — A tongue displaying deep red fissures often indicates a lack of niacin or niacinamide.

Spider Bite — Make a paste out of salt and baking soda mixed with a little water and apply it to the bite.

Stabilized Oxygen — Take five to ten Stabilized Oxygen drops in a glass of water twice a day to supply oxygen to every cell. Next best thing to the Hyperbaric Oxygen Therapy. No awful taste with Stabilized Oxygen drops as in Food Grade Hydrogen Peroxide. Increased dosage up to twenty to fifty drops twice a day is excellent to ward off or heal flu, and to destroy candida fungus infection. But don't extend increased dosage beyond three days. Write to Aerobic Life Products, Inc. (address elsewhere) to obtain the name of a distributor in your area and to obtain full information as to proper intake.

Suma or Pfaffia Paniculata — has been called a cure-all. It comes from the root of a plant called paratoda, which means "for all things." The natives of South America know it to be a blood purifier, an aphrodisiac, a tonic that is a source of energy, and an immunal stimulant. It's an herb tablet which health stores carry under the brand name of *Suma*. Or ask for Suma D'Arco, a tablet combining Suma with Pau D'Arco inner bark of Tabebuia tree. Michael offers an excellent choice!

Sunburn — In severe cases, apply pure Tea Tree Oil. For minor cases dilute oil with cream or baby oil.

Swollen Feet and Legs — Sluggish functioning of the kidneys always shows up in swollen feet and legs. But this reaction can also be stimulated by problems of the heart and liver. Or fat deposits in the legs. Or the retention of salt and water. Try herbal remedies, such as buchu, watermelon seed tea, uva ursa, juniper berries, cranberry juice or tablets. Or try the tablet called "Water Pill" which may be purchased from your health store. It's an all natural herbal diuretic containing a combination of buchu leaves, uva ursa leaves, parsley leaves, juniper berries plus potassium. Or an herb capsule called *PR*, formulated by Dr. John Christopher.

Swollen Glands — Apply a mashed raw tomato poultice as described under *Brain Tumor*. Also increase vitamin C.

Tea Tree Oil — A tree grows in the Australian bush country that possesses miraculous healing powers in its precious oils. It is called the Tea Tree and its oil can heal infections, warts, burns, acne, cold sores, gingivitis, diaper rash, impetigo, lice, ticks and flea infestation, cuts and abrasions, vaginal itching, fungus infection, and ease the pain of arthritis — just to name a few of its many uses. The oil can be taken both internally and externally. It is a safe and pure germicide and disinfectant.

The Tea Tree grows only in Australia and only one of its many varieties possess these wondrous curative properties — the Melaleuca alternifolia. It is important to use only the highest quality Tea Tree Oil and to be sure it is from the proper variety of tree. Do not accept a substitute because it will not give you the same results. It is well worth the added expense.

If you want to learn more about this wonderful gift from God read Sir Jason Winters book, *Breakthrough* or write to B.J. Thomas Products, Inc. To order Tea Tree Oil direct, write to Tri-Sun International, Inc. The addresses are in the last chapter. Winters warns that many are now selling impure or diluted Tea Oil. He urges caution and suggests ordering it from Tri-Sun.

Toxemia — A toxic condition is always aided by sulfur. Buy Oxyquiniline Homeopathic tablets from a homeopathic pharmacy near you or order from Standard Pharmacy (address elsewhere).

Vinegar-Honey Cocktail — Mix two teaspoons of apple cider vinegar and two teaspoons of raw natural honey in a cup of water if your urine test with nitrizine paper indicates alkalinity. Drink from one to four cups a day. It's good for keeping your system acid. It's also good to counteract arthritis. But do be aware it leaches calcium from the body. So don't take more than one cup a day regularly except for arthritic deposits. Even then, make sure you are taking a good source of calcium or, preferably, silica and magnesium.

Vitamin E — has been called the fountain of youth. Its benefits are enormous, such as improved circulation, lowered blood pressure, dissolution of blood clots. It also heals burns, removes scars, relieves premenstrual pain, alleviates leg cramps, stimulates the sex drive, and possesses other advantages too numerous to mention. But see your doctor before making it part of your supplementary approach. Use caution if you suffer from an overactive thyroid, high blood pressure, diabetes, rheumatic heart disease, or if vitamin E decreases the flexibility of lipoprotein, the molecules that carry cholesterol in the bloodstream. Vitamin E sometimes does this, which means lipoproteins are more likely to deposit cholesterol on artery walls. If this is true in your case avoid taking high doses of vitamin E supplements. See your doctor for advice.

The Magic of Walking — Walking is probably the finest exercise there is. Its record for healing is unparalleled. It's now recognized as a method to lose weight and reduce high blood pressure. Other benefits are too numerous to mention.

Whooping Cough — Add vitamin B6 to the diet.

Wounds — Wounds that will not heal require a vitamin C dietary supplement. Apply Aloe Vera gel. Or an ointment called *Pinxav* (Pink Salve), ordered from Harris Wholesale, (address elsewhere). Pinxav was a "regular" on Mama's medicine shelf when we were growing up. And it healed many a wound and sore. It even now occupies a prominent place in my own medicine cabinet. It has healed many a problem when all else failed, even a prescription medicine — for hemorrhoids, for instance. So much so, I now reach for it first for almost anything. It's one of those "old fashioned" formulas, and it works like magic.

Sores and wounds that will not heal could also indicate a lack of sulfur. Ask your druggist or health store for an ointment containing sulfur. Or order sulfur powder and calendula ointment from Standard Homeopathic Pharmacy. Mix together and apply to wound. Dr. Som healed many wounds thusly. Honey is also good for healing wounds and burns.

The Wonders of Zinc — We have long known zinc is important in maintaining the health of the *prostate* gland in men, as well as stimulating the entire reproductive system. As men near middle age the zinc level in their systems seems to diminish, often resulting in inflammations and abnormal functionings of the prostate gland. The sperm count declines and the sex organs may shrink. Zinc is effective in correcting these problems.

Zinc stimulates the entire *immune system*, including aiding the body to produce antibodies which fight foreign invaders. It prevents inflammation of the connective tissues, such as occurs in *rheumatoid arthritis*. It stimulates the flow of enzymes in the digestive system that breaks down food. It promotes the healing of wounds and stimulates muscle contractions. It aids in clearing *acne*. It even prevents *cancer* of the esophagus and bronchial tubes. Lack of zinc can cause the loss of taste and smell, and fingernails that crack, peel or display white spots. The lack is also suspected in cases of anorexia nervosa.

Zinc cannot be absorbed without the presence of picolinic acid. An excellent source of absorbable zinc is *Zinc Picolinate Plus*, available through Swanson's Products. (Address elsewhere.) Do add zinc supplements to your diet if you are experiencing any of these problems. The usual proper dosage is from 15 to 50 milligrams a day. Consult your doctor before beginning such therapy because in certain patients zinc can cause heart problems and anemia.

Zinc Therapy and Blindness — Zinc supplements are now being used to prevent vision loss through the deterioration of the retina, which is the leading cause of eye problems and blindness in the elderly (macular degeneration). Zinc not only slows the eye damage, but often reverses the loss of vision. Laser treatment is sometimes used, but zinc therapy is preferred.

Zinc and Body Odor — Taking zinc tablets daily has proven effective in combating body odor. Be sure the potency isn't over 50 milligrams. Higher doses are toxic.

Potentially Dangerous Substances

Antibiotics — Avoid antibiotics when possible. They usually contain a chemical selected deliberately for its ability to destroy a certain bacteria, but it destroys both good and bad bacteria. Not only are all malevolent and beneficial microbes destroyed, but such drastic medication strips the walls of the intestines of its protective villi, leaving the raw walls exposed to acids, alkalines, painful inflammation, irritations, gases, and the toxins of undigested foods.

It may require weeks or even months for the body to completely recover from the shock of antibiotics. Instead, why not try garlic, a natural antibiotic. It's available in odorless form so it isn't offensive. Why not take it as a daily supplement along with your vitamin program to assure the daily destruction of bad bacteria and exposures to various viruses? If you *must* take an antibiotic, however, never take it without simultaneously taking an acidophilus tablet to assure the daily restoration of good bacteria in the intestines and colon. Many take an acidophilus tablet daily anyway, for safe assurance.

Metals — Everyone knows not to use aluminum cooking pots and pans because the metal sloughs off in your food. It should also be avoided in antacids, deodorants, antiperspirants, and even in the use of foil wrapping paper. *Aluminum is now suspected of being the culprit connected with Alzheimer's and other mental problems.* Unusually high concentrations of aluminum have been found in the brain tissue of victims of *Alzheimer's disease*.

Five patients with memory problems were all found to have had long-term on-the-job exposure to metal vapors, particularly copper. If these two metals are involved, why not suspect others — such as silver-mercury fillings in your teeth? At any rate, since the fillings are also responsible for many other dread diseases, according to leading dentists, why not have them replaced with nonmetallic composites? You could see a dramatic improvement in your memory.

Both Hanna and Michael offer herbal capsules that expel metal from the system. Write either of them if a blood test or hair analysis reveals you have aluminum, lead, mercury and other metals in the bloodstream. Also consider chelation therapy, which removes metals.

Pesticides — Most of us are now aware of the potential dangers of pesticides used in the growing of our fruits and vegetables. But what can you do if you are unable to grow your own food or obtain organically grown foods? One thing you can do is wash all fresh produce as described in Chapter 17, under "Neutralizing Harmful Negative Energy Fields From Foods."

Plastics — We make much of avoiding aluminum pots and pans but I think we do not know enough about the use of plastics and our food. Researching for these writings I discovered that the foundation ingredients of all plastic is petroleum and formaldehyde, a deadly poison.

After reading this, I also began investigating tests and warnings concerning plastic. One test involved two batches of corn. One was planted in a stew pan of porcelain, the other in a plastic container. The corn in the plastic container failed to respond to loving care, light, and any other of the test conditions. The corn in the porcelain container grew strong and tall.

Several years ago it was clearly proven that plastic nursing bottles were extremely dangerous. Since heating them released from the plastic a deadly poison entering the milk drunk by the infant, they could very well cause serious problems, even death. *Could this be the cause of crib deaths?*

If you ever experience blood in the urine check your kitchen utensils carefully to see if you may not be using a plastic utensil in your cooking which could be releasing formaldehyde when heated. Tests revealed that, in some way, the poisons in plastic are released under impact of water, especially heated water, resulting in frightfully poisoned foods. How about the plastic cup from which we drink so much water? And hot coffee? And hot soup?

Dentists interviewed concerning plastic dentures and fillings relate various experiences. One dentist states, "I regard this plastic in the mouth with suspicion. These new plastic dentures and fillings make many of my patients sick. I coat the dentures now with a varnish and this temporarily insulates the plastic from the mouth. It wears off gradually and some folks get used to it." How about all those who don't "get used to it?"

We now use plastic in many things in our kitchen including milk containers, water bottles, food blenders, food storage containers. We use them blindly and in good faith that these items were tested before being released to an unsuspecting public. But practical daily use implies otherwise. Do try to avoid using food or water from heated plastic, such as drinking hot coffee from a plastic cup. And do avoid plastic dental fillings.

Sulfa Drugs — It is not necessary to take sulfa drugs to kill bacteria. They result in dreadful side effects, such as anemia, extreme fatigue and kidney-bladder damage. Take PABA instead. It performs the same function — killing deadly bacteria without the dreaded side effects. Because PABA is so powerful the FDA regulates it by not allowing any food supplement to contain more than 30 milligrams without prescription.

Old fashioned powdered sulfur (not sulfa!) is excellent to kill bacteria and infection. It has nothing to do with sulfa drugs. It's a natural remedy. Purchase it from Standard Homeopathic Pharmacy in powder form or in tiny tablet form called Oxyquiniline. Dissolved (3 tablets) in a glass of water, the solution is great as a gargle for sore throat, or swallowed to kill intestinal bacteria. Use it as a poultice on exterior sores and ulcers.

Wine and Arsenic — Did you know that California wines often contain a dangerous level of arsenic? California Pink Chablis often contains far more than a safe level while some California burgundies, rosés, ports and vermouths contain lesser but still high concentrations. Where is it coming from? It is speculated to be coming from the arsenical pesticides that permeated the soil extensively in California grape fields until 1974. So if you are a wine drinker don't focus steadily on California wines. Alternate with wines from other states or other countries where the residue from pesticides may not be so potent.

Forever Young, a spin-off of this book, suggests using humidifiers and vaporizers. However, I now feel it advisable to strongly caution you regarding their use. Humidifiers and vaporizers can be dangerous because it is impossible to keep them free of bacteria, which may cause pseudomonas in the lungs. Pseudomonas is an extremely difficult bacteria to destroy and the coughing it causes can create additional problems.

Chapter Nineteen

Health Forum — the Conventional Approach

Since many readers have sent me articles on health and healing through the years it seems fitting that I now share this ingathered wisdom. If any suggestion applies to a current problem you're experiencing perhaps this chapter will be helpful. Many items will be mentioned, and in the last chapter you'll be told where the product may be purchased and from whom.

Alzheimer's — is *not* senility. Senility causes minor memory difficulties. Alzheimer's is a gradual loss of almost all memory faculties due to degeneration of nerve endings primarily in the cerebral cortex. Other diseases exhibit similar symptoms, including meningitis, brain tumor, depression, thyroid imbalances, syphilis, even AIDS. In the first stages the patient experiences memory failure of recent events. Gradually he/she becomes more and more confused, exhibits impaired judgment, disorientation, a change in personality, hostility, suspicions. The disease usually lasts from five to eight years. The final stage often requires constant care. Patients cannot feed themselves, can't walk, they stop speaking, they cease to recognize anyone. No cure has yet been found. The drug *THA* has been found helpful. It slows the loss of a brain chemical necessary for memory.

Some dentists who disapprove of silver dental fillings firmly believe the mercury in silver fillings could be a contributing cause for this unfortunate disease. See Chapter 15 if you're interested in checking this information further. And certainly the use of aluminum in cooking and drug and food items is strongly suspected as a contributing factor. Do consider chelation therapy or taking herbal chelation tablets to remove metal from your bloodstream.

One very remarkable gentleman who was diagnosed in 1983 as having Alzheimer's has written a book entitled *Beating Alzheimer's*. When given the devastating news he refused to accept it, even though at the time he couldn't even remember his own phone number and could barely tie his own shoes. Suspecting allergic reactions to foods, chemicals, and pollens, he changed his entire living and eating habits. In April of 1987 a brain scan showed no trace of Alzheimer's. If you wish to read this informative and encouraging book write to the Alzheimer's Treatment, Research and Education Foundation (address in Chapter 20). Also write Hanna Kroeger who has published a booklet offering natural aids.

Blood Saving Treatment to Avoid Amputations — Dr. David Knighton, director of the wound healing clinic at the University of Minnesota, reports that his research group has discovered a method of saving a wounded leg from amputation. The method is to remove a small amount of the patient's blood and, in a laboratory, remove the blood platelets. The platelets are that part of the blood which contain essential healing substances. Each day the patient applies the platelet-rich formula of his own blood to the wound. It's left for 12 hours and then removed. Enough blood is drawn to create enough formula for 10 to 12 weeks of application. The wound is usually completely healed by that time.

This treatment heals the deepest kind of skin ulcers usually in about ten weeks. Amputations are prevented in 85% of the cases. This treatment will aid diabetics suffering from non-healing diabetic skin ulcers and prevent amputation of their feet or legs. It will also heal nonhealing pressure sores that result from being bedridden or confined to a wheelchair. It will also heal leg and foot ulcers due to diseased blood vessels. It truly appears to be a miracle treatment. And the good part is that it is done by using the patient's own blood. Doctors interested in prescribing it for their patients should call Dr. Knighton at his clinic — (612) 626-6666.

A firm called CuraTech Inc. may also be contacted for information concerning this procedure. Their number is (516) 231-8680. All researchers and doctors involved in this new discovery declare it to be a major breakthrough and that it will certainly save many patients from undergoing amputations of wounded limbs.

The first known leg transplant has occurred at an East German hospital near Berlin. It was a complete success according to Dr. Hartwig Meissner, chief of staff. Perhaps more will take place, affording life-changing consequences to unfortunate patients who lose limbs.

Anesthetics — A new anesthetic called *Propofal* enables the patient to revive about seven minutes after surgery and it has less severe side effects than other anesthetics.

Anesthetics with Lollipops — "Lollipops" laced with pre-surgery anesthetics are now offered to children to avoid the use of the frightening and painful needle. The anesthetic works fast because it enters the bloodstream through the sensitive tissues inside the mouth, directly affecting the brain and bypassing the liver.

The Magic of Aspirin — We've mentioned the value of aspirin to prevent heart attacks in Chapter 10 and again in Chapter 18 regarding the immune system. Aspirin, of course, is the leading tablet for all types of headaches, toothaches, muscular aches, arthritis pain and for reducing fever. It counteracts swelling and lowers blood sugar levels to reduce the possibility of diabetes. It is being tested as a preventive of cataracts. Later, more will be said under *Senility* regarding aspirin as an aid to mental problems.

However, a word of warning is in order here. . . do not give aspirin to children under the age of 18 who have a flu virus. Aspirin combined with the flu virus can cause life threatening Reye's syndrome in children. It should be avoided by people with ulcers, kidney damage or liver disease because of its blood thinning activity. It should never be given to hemophiliacs.

If you find it necessary to take aspirin often, as in the case of arthritis, or for heart problems, do be aware that small bleeding in the gastrointestinal tract could lead to iron depletion. Discuss with your doctor the possibility of needing an iron supplement. You might also need folic acid and vitamin C. Increase the intake of both if you are a long-time aspirin user. Daily intake may be "overkill." Every other day seems more advisable even to prevent heart problems.

Asthma — is now being helped by a new drug called

Azmacort. Although it *is* a drug it's a considerable improvement over prednisone, a drug which produces unpleasant side effects. And try vitamin B6. It's reputed to be effective in preventing attacks. *Cromolyn sodium*, an experimental drug used to treat asthma, also may be found useful to protect the lining of the lungs against the effects of smog, vehicle exhaust and cigarette smoke.

There is now available a lightweight device for home use called *Fisoneb* to aid those with asthma, bronchitis, emphysema, cystic fibrosis and pneumonia. The unit breaks drugs down into a fine aerosol mist which can be inbreathed during sleep. Use in the home prevents hospitalization for chronic patients.

Another new drug, called *Uniphyl*, is useful in reducing the severity of asthma attacks during the night, when many asthma patients wake up coughing, wheezing and experiencing extreme difficulty in breathing because the air passages tend to shrink at night. The slow release properties of Uniphyl make it an excellent choice for night use in controlling asthma. It should be taken at the evening meal because its effectiveness peaks between 4 a.m. and 6 a.m., which is the time asthmatics most need the medication.

Healing Bandages — New bandages are called *Bubble Bandages* — because a bubble of natural body fluid forms beneath them — allow healing oxygen to enter a wound, keeping moisture in but sealing harmful bacteria out. The new bandages, which resemble clear plastic food wrap, significantly reduce healing time. They also eliminate pain. These new bandages are made of polyurethane. They are superior to other bandages because, should infection develop, doctors can discern it right away through the clear plastic bubble. These bandages are used on such wounds as scrapes, light burns, removal of skin for grafts and closed surgical incisions. Seek for them in the department which sells Band-Aid dressings.

Electric Bandages — Speaking of bandages, Dr. Richard Bentall, of Bioelectronics Corp. in Washington, DC, reports that he and his aides are developing an amazing new electric bandage to replace gauze dressings. His electric bandage will use radio waves to pump electromagnetic energy into the skin to speed healing cuts, wounds, and surgical incisions. The wrist watch-sized device improves healing by reducing swelling and inflammation.

Bed-wetting — Vitamin B6 should aid in overcoming this problem. Also ask your doctor about a drug called *Amitriptylene*. It's reported to aid in bed-wetting. Also to aid in bladder incontinence for adults. But use it only as a last resort. It has some unpleasant side effects, such as dry mouth.

Blood Transfusions — When one is facing surgery of any kind it is often suggested that you visit the hospital and have your own blood drawn to be used during the surgical procedure in the event you need a blood transfusion. This seems a simple answer to avoiding blood from another person, either on moral grounds or to avoid the possibility of infection.

Now comes news of a recycling machine that allows your own blood to be used during the procedure of surgery. The blood normally lost during surgery is saved and passed through the new device — first through a filter which removes the heaviest particles, then through a centrifuge, which separates damaged and unwanted debris, leaving the blood clean and pure. Thus the doctor can return the patient's own blood if blood is needed. If you are facing surgery do inquire concerning this recycling machine from your doctor.

Artificial Blood — A group of researchers working in Irvine, California, announced that they have invented artificial blood. It is produced, they say, by cleaning up red blood cells taken from mammals (animals) to rid it of infectious disease, then "gluing" back molecules of hemoglobin on a large scale for the resulting substance. It has not yet gained approval from the FDA. Once it is released it will be called *Oxy-Gen*. With the current fear about deadly AIDS, such an invention may be remarkable in lifesaving situations. The group of researchers failed to mention what type of mammals were used in their experiments.

It should be remembered, however, that many animals have been fed hormones to induce weight gain and fats. They have also been fed other substances in their diet. It is to be hoped that the blood cleaning process destroys more than infectious disease before it is used on humans.

Body Building — At last our FDA is recognizing the technique of building strong muscles through rapid-pulsating electric currents. The Russians have been using electric shock treatment for years. The current contracts and releases muscles, performing via electricity what we do by isometrics — tensing and releasing muscles. This surely will encourage our would-be athletes to cease their use of deadly steroids and turn to this more natural means of muscle development.

Don't resort to raw eggs for strength. They contain a protein which blocks the immune system's ability to absorb biotin, a B vitamin vital for normal growth. Biotin is also necessary to utilize fats, protein and carbohydrates.

Burn Treatment — Dr. Bruce Achauer, director of the

University of California's Burn Center at Irvine, near Los Angeles, reports that *Cyclosporine*, the drug that makes organ transplants successful, is now being used to halt the rejection of cadaver skin grafted onto severely burned people. Dr. A. Richard Grossman, director of California's Sherman Oaks Burn Center, agrees, stating: "While cadaver skin has been employed for some time as a temporary covering for some burns, we are using cadaver skin as a permanent replacement in some cases" — such as when a patient has lost too much of his/her own skin to be left for grafting — "without the cadaver skin grafts, these patients would have died." Cyclosporine aids such patients to accept the cadaver skin graft. The drug can be discontinued after a few months.

Canker Sores — A new over-the-counter medicine called *Zilactin* far excels other drugs in healing painful canker sores. It is effective for hours compared to only a few moments for other remedies. It's a gel-like ointment applied directly on the mouth ulcer. It forms a tough film that covers the ulcer, protecting it from foods, drinks and other irritations. Canker sores can also be helped greatly or even healed by sucking an antacid tablet — Pepto Bismol, Tums, Rolaids, Maalox Plus. The tablet will break down the mouth acids, which may have caused the canker sore in the first place.

Circumcision — If you insist on circumcising your male infant, though some medical authorities consider it unnecessary, extremely painful, and traumatic, there now appears to be a procedure to reduce the pain and the trauma. It's called a *dorsal penile nerve block*, an almost painless injection just prior to circumcision. The anesthetic is totally safe and certainly affords the infant a measure of mercy. Ask your doctor about it.

Cold Sores — For cold sores try *Carmex*. It's been around a long time, and many people swear by it. Purchase at drug store or order through the Vermont Country Store. (Address in last chapter.)

Coma Patients — Patients who have overdosed on tranquilizers such as Valium and Atavan are being restored to consciousness through a new drug which is injected into the vein. It is also being used as a post-surgical aid to regaining consciousness when difficulty is experienced. It's called *Flumazenil*. The drug quickly reaches the brain and instantly awakens the comatose patient. The new drug is expected to benefit thousands of people and save many lives.

Diabetes — A new report states that specialists may soon be able to detect diabetes up to seven years before it even starts. Researchers at the Joslin Diabetes Center have detected an abnormal protein in the blood, called the *64K antibody*, which apparently triggers diabetes, or signals its approach. They hope that destroying the antibody can prevent diabetes from ever developing. It at least offers an opportunity to begin effective treatment to hopefully ward off the disease.

A new device called the *Diacare System* offers tremendous aid to diabetics. It's a hand-held computer which instantly and accurately tells the patient how much insulin is necessary for daily injections. It reveals blood sugar levels and analyzes food intake, saving the diabetic the necessity of evaluating complicated formulas.

Portable insulin pumps are now available which enable diabetics to regulate insulin injections. Laser therapy is now preventing diabetics from becoming blind. Implantable artificial devices that mimic the natural function of the pancreas are now being perfected. Researchers are also working to develop means to prevent the immune system's destruction of the cells of the pancreas which destroy the ability of the pancreas to produce insulin. For more information on diabetes, see the last chapter for the toll-free "hot line" number.

Ears

Ear Infections — Often caused by the bacterium Branhamell catarholis, or B-cat virus, can now be cured by a new antibiotic called *Augmetin*. Ear infection, if untreated, can lead to permanent hearing damage. Be cautious about having tubes put in your child's ears. Research has found delicate surgery is often unnecessary. Antibiotics often work as well.

New Age Hearing Aids — A computerized tiny hearing aid which consists of two chips no larger than an aspirin will soon revolutionize the hearing aid industry. It's called a *Digital Aid* produced by 3-M Corporation. One can wear it inside or outside the ear. And it will pick up lower and higher frequency noises which the present type cannot comfortably accommodate. But there is now available a new device called a *Zeta Noise Blocker* that reduces background sounds while still amplifying voices. It's a computer chip which monitors frequencies of sounds coming into the hearing aid, then reduces noises such as traffic, air conditioning, lawn mowers and crowd noises.

A new drug known as *Ginkgo Biloba* is proving extremely beneficial to the deaf. Made from the dried leaves of a Japanese tree, the Ginkgo, it is marketed in West Germany under the name of *Rockan* or *Tebonin*. In tests one in four patients regained their hearing completely. Others reported obvious improvement. In many cases tinnitus —

ringing in the ear — totally disappeared. It's not yet available in the U.S. but patients may ask their doctor to fill out a special "Compassionate IND" form to gain FDA approval. The drug works by improving blood circulation throughout the body and is especially beneficial to those whose hearing loss is caused by a blood flow problem in the ear.

Epilepsy — If you are an epileptic you may be interested in a new study which reveals that two-thirds of patients studied were able to give up their medication if given smaller and smaller dosages in a withdrawal plan. Discovering they were free of seizures came as a distinct surprise to these patients. It was found that a gradual withdrawal was necessary in order for the experiment to be successful. See your doctor for details.

Eyes

Contact Lenses — saturated with medication are now available which release medication over a period of from eight hours to three days. Then the lenses dissolve. Also available are implantable tablets that gradually dissolve, releasing medication via time-release. There are also eye droppers with smaller tips which prevent overflow and waste.

Ophthalmologists tell us that while wearing contact lenses that change the color of your eyes is not harmful they *can* cause some problems. A new study shows that the tinted band of opaque color dots can slide over part of the pupil, causing some loss of peripheral vision. The problem can be alleviated somewhat by proper fitting.

Eye Transplants — Surgeons at a research facility outside Sao Paulo, Brazil, are now removing the eyes from donor corpses and transplanting them into the blind. This technique replaces the usual procedure of corneal transplant as it replaces the entire eye. They report fantastic results. The transplant must be done immediately after the death of the donor. Eye specialists worldwide are watching these new developments with keen interest. If they prove successful it could mean the end of blindness or even diseased eyes for the human race.

Glaucoma — Good news for those with glaucoma. There's a new ten-minute surgical procedure which can save eyesight. It's called *internal sclerectomy*. The new procedure won't restore vision already lost but it will halt the progress of the disease immediately. So says Dr. Ray Brown, director of the glaucoma service at the Emory University Eye Clinic in Atlanta, Georgia.

Laser for Eye Defects — Summit Technology of Watertown, Massachusetts, reports that researchers, using an amazing new "cold" laser which they manufacture, are reshaping the human eye to correct vision defects. The device treats astigmatism, nearsightedness, farsightedness, cataracts and glaucoma. Summit Technology sincerely believes this laser device will eventually make eyeglasses obsolete.

Pinkeye (Conjuctivitis) — is an inflammation of the filmy membrane covering the white of the eye. When this membrane becomes inflamed the blood vessels enlarge and redden — thus the name "pinkeye." Itching, pain, and/or discharge may accompany the redness. The inflammation can be caused by bacterial infections, viruses, allergies, contact lenses, smoke, chemicals in eye make-up, chlorine in swimming pools, or an injury to the eye. The treatment depends on the cause. It is best to see a doctor to determine the cause and treatment since, untreated, it can lead to serious problems. It is extremely contagious if caused by a virus or bacteria and all sanitary precautions should be taken.

Fever Finder — New on the market is a thermometer that is computerized. It's called First-Temp. The probe is inserted in the ear or even touched to the outer ear, and your temperature registers in only a few seconds. Thank goodness! I could die of a fever before I could ever read the gauge on a regular thermometer. At last there's a simple temperature finder for simpletons like me.

Gallstones — A new technique for removal seems imminent. It involves inserting a catheter with a tiny plastic bag on the end into the gallbladder. When the bag has scooped up the stone, a sonar wave then blasts it to miniature pieces, which the body can then painlessly eliminate. A new drug, *Ursodiol,* is also now being used to combat gallstones. Removal of the gallbladder has until now been the usual procedure. The new drug has few if any side effects. It is marketed under the name of *Actigall* in pill form which dissolves the stones, enabling the debris to be naturally eliminated from the body.

Herpes — Laser beams are now being used against the pain and discomfort of genital herpes. When used on patients during the disease's early stages the laser treatment prevents herpes from recurring. The treatment, usually painless, can be done in a doctor's office. Millions of Americans suffer from this sexually transmitted disease which causes sores to appear periodically on the genitals. The laser treatment offers immediate relief from pain. The laser beam literally kills the virus and usually it does not reoccur. Doctors seeking more information about this treatment are advised to contact Dr. Robert Scott, assistant clinical professor of obstetrics and gynecology at the University of Southern California in Los Angeles.

Oral Herpes and Toothbrushes — Researchers at the University of Oklahoma have found that discarding your toothbrush often could prevent a chain reaction of breakouts. A toothbrush, constantly a moist environment, can harbor the virus for up to seven days, infecting and reinfecting the lips and the entire mouth. It doesn't help to disinfect the toothbrush. It stays infected. The three different times the brush should be discarded are: during the prodrome, or tingly, phase which signals a breakout; when the blister breaks; and as soon as the blister is gone.

But herpes or not, the toothbrush should be discarded for a new one every two or three weeks. Even under the healthiest conditions, it breeds bacteria. The latest report advises that your toothbrush should not be kept in the bathroom because each time the commode is flushed germs and bacteria invade the atmosphere. Seeking a moist environment, the toothbrush becomes a haven. So keep it in the bedroom within reach of the bathroom. Or buy an enclosed container for toothbrushes.

For both genital and oral herpes there is a drug called *Acyclovir* which may be helpful. But the treatment is quite expensive. I'm not enough familiar with it to mention side effects. See your doctor.

Hiccups — can now be controlled with a new drug called *Baclofen*, which stimulates the production of a brain chemical responsible for stopping nerve impulses from stimulating the diaphragm, which causes hiccups.

Impetigo — Impetigo is a skin problem which begins with tiny blisters forming on the skin which gradually become covered by a thick crust. The blisters spread to other areas and the itching can be agonizing. Often the arms, legs and face are affected. Most of the antibiotic ointments used in the past have caused cramps, vomiting and diarrhea. A new ointment has just come on the market called *Bactroban* which acts as a two-in-one treatment. It is a prescription drug but is extremely effective in relieving the itching and healing the blisters, preventing their spread to other areas. But use no longer than absolutely necessary — it may contain sulfa drugs damaging to the kidneys. Or try cold pressed castor oil or Tea Tree oil.

Leukemia — The drug *Asparatimase* is often used to control acute lymphoblastic leukemia. But some children reject it because their immune systems attack it. Scientists have now discovered a way to "hide" the drug by attaching it to a harmless molecule, allowing it to circulate through the body for longer periods. This enhances the effectiveness of the drug so that the immune system of the child has an opportunity to improve enough to fight the leukemia.

Medical Information — A new book, "*Dial 800 for Health*," published by The People's Medical Society, provides toll free phone numbers which you may call to have an expert answer your questions concerning health. The information is free. To obtain the book send $4.00 to: The People's Medical Society. (Address in last chapter.)

Multiple Sclerosis — A drug often prescribed for flu has been found helpful for MS patients. It's call *Amantadine*. Removal of silver dental fillings is resulting in recovery of MS. See Chapter 15 for the correct procedure in removing fillings.

Muscle Spasms — Are often brought under control by taking silica herbal tablets (horsetail) which are beginning to be recognized as a superior means of supplying calcium to the system. Whereas calcium often creates calcification and arthritis, silica does not. Vitamin B6 is extremely beneficial. On the drug approach for severe spasms a drug called *Botulinum Toxin* is reducing the distress of many patients. It's injected directly into a constricted muscle.

There is another treatment now being used that has been quite successful. Low doses of a drug called *Sinemet*, which has been used in heavier doses to treat Parkinson's disease since 1975, is now being given to people who suffer from "restless leg syndrome," a chronic condition that causes a crawling sensation deep inside their legs, or triggers spasms that make their legs jerk when they try to sleep. For some, with severe cases, the improvement has changed their lives.

Parkinson's Disease — Doctors in Stockholm, Sweden, are performing an operation which implants tissue from the adrenal gland into the brain center which produces dopamine, a brain substance disrupted by the disease. The brain center then begins to produce a natural supply of dopamine, creating dramatic improvement in the patients. But the breakthrough is still very experimental.

Dentists who advocate the removal of silver fillings from the teeth insists that patients with Parkinson's have greatly benefited by the removal of such fillings which may affect the brain center which produces dopamine. In tests, vitamins C and E have proven beneficial in the early stages of the disease. Their use delays the necessity of beginning the standard drug treatment. There is also a promising new drug called *Permax*.

Polio — Many polio victims suffer post-polio syndrome (PPS), including muscle weakness and breathing problems. For the latest information for help write to the address given in the last chapter, under PPS.

Rosacea — an adult form of acne, is the disease that caused W. C. Fields to have a big red nose. The disease affects adults in their 30s and 40s, many of whom are not even aware that it is treatable. A new drug, *MetroGel*, which cures rosacea is now available by prescription, so see your doctor if you are afflicted with this disease. Or try the garlic poultice mentioned in Chapter 11 regarding cancer.

Senility — Researchers are discovering *aspirin* to be effective in bringing about a significant change in the elderly who suffer from a form of senility called multi-infarct dementia. So says a report from Dr. John S. Meyer of Baylor College of Medicine in Houston, Texas. It has been found to reverse absent-mindedness, memory loss and behavioral deterioration suffered by 30% of senile patients.

The disease, caused by tiny blood clots inside the head, is apparently stabilized by aspirin which increases blood flow inside the brain. Dr. Meyer gave his treated group of patients an aspirin a day. Their improvement, as compared to his nontreated patients, was so obvious that after three years he ceased the testing, feeling the test to be unfair to those not receiving the daily aspirin.

Research also shows that as we age our absorption of vitamin B6 changes dramatically, reports Dr. Robert M. Russell of Tufts University's Schools of Medicine and Nutrition. Insufficient levels of vitamin B6 can cause reduced brain activity so older people should increase their daily intake.

Steroids — Steroids have proven to be so dangerous they should no longer be considered either by athletes or anyone else. Amino acid supplements have been found to produce identical effects, so why not choose the natural approach that of amino acids? Steroids produce major health problems while amino acids produce immuno-stimulants.

The health hazards include the effect upon the reproductive system, the cardiovascular system, the liver, and the glandular system. Since they affect the glandular system the manufacture of naturally occurring hormones is affected. When steroids are taken the synthetic hormones in the bloodstream cause the pituitary to cease distributing its own testosterone production resulting in low sperm count and possible sterility. Effects upon the liver include cancer, peliosis, hepatitis, and impaired liver function.

Tremors — There's a new drug called *Primidone* which is being used successfully to combat tremors. For full information contact Dr. William Koller, International Tremor Foundation, Box E, 360 W. Superior St., Chicago, IL 60610.

Ulcers — Surprisingly, *Pepto-Bismol* is better medicine for ulcers than the drug *Cimetidine*. Tests have proven that Pepto-Bismol, generically known as bismuth subsalicitate, is not only good to seal ulcers and protect them from painful acids, but is also excellent for diarrhea.

Time was when everybody, doctors included, thought ulcers were the result of stress. They called them the executive syndrome. But they know now that isn't true, nor is a bland diet suggested. Milk was once thought to be the leading curative or "reliefant" but that couldn't possibly be true since milk calcium triggers an increase in acids — and acids are to be avoided. A change in diet may certainly be indicated in that you should no longer eat the hot foods you previously enjoyed. Not hot in a heat sense but hot in a seasoning sense.

It might be wise to switch to a vegetarian diet, even if it is only temporary, because meat contains much uric acid. It would be wise to give up smoking because tobacco interrupts the flow of blood to the stomach, interfering with basic utilization. The action of protein in the stomach produces acid which is a major reason for reducing your intake of meats. Ulcers, like a young man's fancy, seem to flare up in the spring. But strangely enough, the flare up is repeated in the autumn. It shouldn't require much time to discover which foods cause you discomfort. Eliminate them from your diet. Surely you must eliminate caffeine, alcohol and tobacco, all of which stimulate acid secretions.

A new ulcer drug, *Pepcid*, is proving extremely effective in reducing or relieving the pain of ulcers. Many prefer it to *Tagamet* or *Zantac*. Pepcid enables the patient to return to a fairly normal diet without fear of painful, burning sensations or stomach cramps. A drug called *Cytotec* helps prevent ulcers in those patients who find it necessary to take aspirin or *Naprosyn*, which are often prescribed for arthritis. All these ulcer drugs have unpleasant side effects.

Another new drug is *Axid* — it's cheaper and extremely safe. Taken once a day at bedtime ulcers heal in about three-fourths of patients in four weeks. So says Dr. Maurice A. Cerulli, assistant professor of medicine at State University in New York. Tested on 5,000 people, it had no serious side effects. Nor did it interfere with other drugs the patient needed. Taken at bedtime it inhibits gastric acid secretions during sleep when damage to the walls of the stomach and intestines most often occurs. Axid eliminates peptic ulcer pain in only a few days. Another new drug is *Omeprazole*. It has been found much more effective than conventional ulcer drugs.

But, again, the good old stand-by Pepto-Bismol seems to rank as a leading healer and it has no side effects. Why not try it at bedtime and see if a healing occurs?

Willpower — a drug called *Fluoxetine-Hydrochloride* is being called a "willpower pill," because it suppresses the appetite, which aids in reducing programs, and it also curbs the desire for heavy drinking.

Chapter Twenty

Health Products

I promised to tell you more about the products I've recommended and where you might order them. Special distributors and products are listed first:

Fanie Products and Distributors:

Karie Hayden or Carlis Orlando, 975 Hornblend #D, San Diego, CA 92109 or P.O. Box 81502, San Diego, CA 92138; 619-581-3321.
Valjean McGinty, Oma Enterprises, P.O. Box 4873, Palm Springs, CA 92264.
Florence Johnson,174-22 Armstrong Ave., Irvine, CA 92714 ***or call*** 1-800-FANI to get the name of the Fanie representative in your area.

Hanna Kroeger, 1122 Pearl St., Boulder, CO 80302; 303-443-0261.

Lesley and Michael Tierra, P.O. Box 712, Santa Cruz, CA 95061; 408-336-8141.

Other Recommended Products and People

Acupuncture: Master Sehan Kim, 3875 Wilshire Blvd, Los Angeles, CA 90010; 213-874-5646.

Acupuncture and Oriental Herbal Remedies: Dr. Timothy Yea, 326 N. Euclid Ave., Upland, CA 91786; 714-946-6444. Northern California; 415-685-8444. Mid-West; 913-648-0283.

Allergy Specialist: Dr. James Privitera, 105 N. Grand view, Covina, CA 91732; 818-966-1618.

AR+: Dynapro International Inc, P.O. Box 3002, Ogden UT 84409.

Bar Magnet: Bio Health Ent. Inc., Rt. 3, Box 121, Murray, KY 42071.

Beating Alzheimer's: The Alzheimer's Treatment and Research Foundation, 2916 Commercial Ave., Ancortes, WA 98221; 1-800-343-1260.

Carmex: Vermont Country Store: Mail Order Office, P.O. Box 3000, Manchester, VT 05255.

Chiropractor's Special Pillow for Sleeping: Dr. Noll Walker, P.O. Box 2052, Upland, CA 91785

Collis-Curve Toothbrush: Sir George Collis, 313 W 48th St., Minneapolis, MN 55409.

Colostrum Cream or Tablets: Dr. Charles Bunner, 124 East F St., Ontario, CA 91764; 714-983-0581.

Comfortably Yours: 61 W. Hunter Ave., Maywood, NJ 07607; 201-368-3499.

Date Sugar: Shields Date Gardens, Indio, CA 92201.

DMSO: Cleveland Clinic, 9500 Euclid Ave., Cleveland, OH 44106.

Earth Force Minerals: B&K Products, 5083 Camelot Dr., Mobile, AL 36619.

Free Medical Information: "Dial 800 for Health," People's

Medical Society, P.O. Box FC, 14 E. Minor St. Emmaus, PA 18049.

Fruit Vegetable Wash: Consumer Health Research, Inc., 8055 Lankersheim Blvd. #9, N. Hollywood, CA 91605.

Health Information Service: P.O. Box 1922, Chula Vista, CA 92012.

Hemorr-ice: Technology 2000 Corp, 325 10th St., Lakewood, NJ 08701.

Holistic Dentists:

Dr. Joel Berger, Bayside, NY; 718-225-2121.

Dr. Hal Huggins, Box 2589, Colorado Springs, CO 80901.

Dr. Mark Hulet, 14201 Kentwood Blvd. #2, Victorville, CA 92392; 619-241-8874.

Dr. Michael Ziff, Orlando, FL; 305-293-3185.

Homeopathic Remedies:

Dr. Edward Bach Center, Mt. Vernon, Sotwell Wallingford, Oxon, OX10, OPZ, England.

Biological Homeopathic Industries, Inc., 11600 Cochiti SE, Albuquerque, NM 87123.

Boericke & Tafel, 1011 Arch St., Philadelphia, PA 19107; 215-922-2967.

Edgar Cayce Products: Cayce Corner, 4018 N. 40th St., Phoenix, AZ 85018; 602-955-0551.

Herbal Home Products, Box 258, Rescue, CA 95672; 916-626-5046.

Similia Laboratories, Inc., 5946 Okeechobee Blvd, W. Palm Beach, FL 33417.

Standard Homeopathic Pharmacy, Box 61067, Los Angeles, CA 90061.

Swanson Health Products: P.O. Box 2803, Fargo, ND 58108; 1-800-437-4148.

Homeopathic Doctors:

American Center For Homeopathy, 7297-H Lee Hwy., Falls Church, VA 22042; 703-534-2600.

National Center For Homeopathy, 1500 Massachusetts Ave. N.W. #41, Washington, DC 20005.

Incontinence: Dr. Paul de Ridder, 1125 E. 17th St., E222, Santa Ana, CA 92701; 714-547-5741 (or) 714-542-3536.

Infertility: American Fertility Society at 1(205)933-8494. **Or** contact Resolve Inc., 5 Water St., Arlington, VA 02174; (617)643-2424.

Laetrile and Tribalene: VitaChem International, 241 Hazel Ave., Redwood City, CA 94061.

Laser Treatments: Dr. Franklin Loffer, St. Joseph's Hospital, 350 W. Thomas Rd., Phoenix, AZ 85013.

Levitor: Kirksville College of Osteopathic Medicine, 800 Jefferson St., Kirksville, MO 63501.

Light Bulb and Tubes:

Kiva-Light, L.O. Anderson Research Laboratory, 5029 Echo St., Los Angeles, CA 90042; 213-254-7169.

Ott Light Systems, Inc., 306 E. Cota St., Santa Barbara, CA 93101.

Lithotripsy: Dr. Glen Preminger, University of Texas - Dallas, Richardson, TX 75080.

Magnetic Mattress Pad: Ruby M. Morrow, 11401 Central Ave. #103, Chino, CA 91710

Mineral Salt and Sweet Charge: The Dews Co., P.O. Box 147, Mineral Wells, TX 76067.

Mixed seeds, goat's milk whey, yeast flakes and other products: Arthur Blackmer, National Fruit and Vegetable Industries, P.O. Box 92643, Pasadena, CA 91109.

National Health Federation: P.O. Box 688, Monrovia, CA 91016.

Neti Pot: Himalayan Institute, RR1, Box 400, Honesdale, PA 18431.

Pinxav (Pink Salve): Harris Wholesale, 30600 Carter St., Solon, OH 44139.

Post Polio Awareness and Support Society: 813 Darwin Ave., Victoria, British Columbia, Canada V8X 2X7.

Real Salt: American Orso, Inc., 75 N. State, Redmund, UT 84652; 801-529-7487.

Rodaquin: S.R. Winslow, P.O. Box 1985, Chula Vista, CA 92012.

Shoe Inserts: Luxis International, Dept. XWW189, 712 N. 34th St., Seattle, WA 98103.

Stabilized Oxygen: Aerobic Life Products, Inc., 9811 Ferguson, Dallas, TX 75228; 214-328-3159 (or) 1-800-798-0707.

Suboccipital Pillow: SPS Distributors, 1545 N. Verdugo Rd., Glendale, CA 91208.

Super Adrenal Formula: BBC, P.O. Box 4125, Oroville, CA 95965.

Tea Tree Oil: Tri-Sun International, Inc., 2700 Chandler, Bldg. A#1, Las Vegas, NV 89120; 702-736-3990 (or) 1-800-447-1616.

For Information: B.J. Thomas Products, Inc., 1164 Bishop St., Suite 124, Honolulu, HI 96813.

TMJ Foundation: 340 Wilshire Blvd. #310, Los Angeles, CA 90010.

Tremors:. Dr. William Koller, International Tremor Foundation, Box E, 360 W. Superior St., Chicago, IL 60610.

Vision Blood Analyzer: Customer Service, Abbott Laboratories, Abbott Park, IL 60064.

White Flower Analgesic Balm: The Trace Co., P.O. Box 2023, Carson City, NV 89702. Or at your health store.

Toll-Free Health Hot Lines:

AIDS: (National AIDS Hot Line) 1-800-342-AIDS.
ALZHEIMER'S DISEASE: (Alzheimer's Association) 1-800-621-0379. In Illinois, 1-800-572-60327.
ARTHRITIS: (Arthritis Foundation) 1-800-283-7800.
Breathing PROBLEMS: 1-800-222-LUNG.
CANCER: (Cancer Information Service) 1-800-4 CANCER.
DIABETES: (American Diabetes Association) 1-800-232-3472.
DRUG PROBLEMS: (National Parents' Rescue Institute for Drug Education — PRIDE) 1-800-241-7946.
EPILEPSY: (Epilepsy Foundation of America) 1-800-EFA-1000. In California, 1-800-572-3330.
GENERAL HEALTH PROBLEMS: (Information Center) 1-800-221-5517.
KIDNEY DISEASE: (American Kidney Fund) 1-800-638-8299.
PHYSICAL and *MENTAL TRAUMA* (American Trauma Society) 1-800-556-7890.
SECOND SURGICAL OPINIONS: (Health Care Financing Administration) 1-800-638-6833.